SEARCHING FOR CENTER

SEARCHING FOR CENTER

A Tai Chi Master's Journey

Master Henry Wang

With

Ted Libby

Littlewood Press

Title: Searching for Center
Subtitle: A Tai Chi Master's Journey
Authors: Henry Wang with Edward M. Libby
Published by: Littlewood Press, Issaquah, WA

First Edition, 2021
Published in the United States of America

ISBN: 978-1-7369978-0-2 (hardcover)
ISBN: 978-1-7369978-1-9 (paperback)
ISBN: 978-1-7369978-2-6 (e-book)

Statement re Errors: Any factual errors, misspellings, incorrect usage of terms, and any other mistakes of any kind or nature are accidental and unintentional. Corrections to future editions will be made upon learning of the same.

Disclaimer and Caution re Exercises: The contents of this book are intended for informational purposes. Undertaking any physical activity, including the internal energy arts such as tai chi and/or chi kung (qi gong), may carry risks of injury or other harm to oneself or others. To reduce any such risks, the reader is advised and cautioned to consult their health care provider or other professional before beginning this or any other martial arts or exercise regimen. The practices and methods described should not be used as a substitute for professional medical diagnosis or treatment.

The author(s) and publisher disclaim any liability for loss, injury, or risk, personal or otherwise, whether occasioned directly or indirectly, from reading, following, using, or misusing any practices, exercises, advice, or lessons contained in the material presented. No written work can replace well-informed, in-person instruction.

Dedication

I dedicate this book to my parents, my wife, and my children.

Henry Wang
(Wang, Hui-Juin)

"Yong Yi, Bu Yong Li"

用意不用力

"Use the Mind, Not Force."

CONTENTS

Introduction:

Since starting on this tai chi journey my ambition has been to constantly improve my understanding of this art and to contribute to its evolution and advancement for the next generation. Having now completed over forty-five years of concentrated study and effort, I want to share what I've learned so that others may benefit from my experience and enjoy a long and healthy life.

I hope that you will be motivated to explore the new and innovative ideas being presented and to experiment with these methods in your tai chi practice. The time spent training in this manner will certainly produce health benefits, rejuvenate the body and spirit, and promote longevity. In addition, for those interested in the self-defense aspects of tai chi, my "Search Center" training regimen can provide an effective response to aggression and do so in a manner that is consistent with the soft way. Sharing this hard-won knowledge with others, particularly the next generation of tai chi students, is my principal reason for writing this book.

Henry Wang
Comox, British Columbia
Canada
2020

SECTION ONE:

MY TAI CHI BACKGROUND

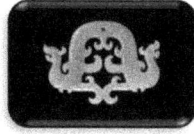

Chapter 1: Starting Out

I AM A STUDENT and teacher of the Chinese martial art Tai Chi Chuan (Taijiquan). I have devoted most of my adult life to improving and conveying my understanding of its underlying Taoist philosophy, its health-giving benefits, and its complex depths as an applied martial art. Although I didn't realize it at the outset, this rather uncommon career would become my life's work. I began my tai chi studies in 1974 and I have made it my principal occupation since 1986. This writing marks over forty-five years since I began my tai chi journey. Throughout it has been a vocation and not just a job. I say that I am a student as well as a teacher because I am still learning. The years have shown me that the study of tai chi is most surely open-ended. The limits of this art are yet unknown. There is always more to explore, more to discover, more to share with my students and the tai chi community at large.

Although I had trained in other martial arts before I took up tai chi, I was already in my early twenties before I had my first series of tai chi lessons. Once exposed to it, I quickly became obsessed with learning all I could. Tai chi became a passionate pursuit and my enthusiasm for the sport motivated me to train intensively each day. The disciplined regimen I undertook enabled me to become increasingly successful in the tai chi tournaments I entered. By the age of twenty-five, I had won the first of my several national championships in tai chi Push Hands (*Tui Shou*) in my native country, Taiwan. A few years later, at the height of those successes and to the surprise of many, I willingly gave up competitive tai chi completely. I did so in the hope of finding a solution to the famous and puzzling paradox from the Tai Chi Classics which proclaims that "four ounces can move a thousand pounds". Can this be true I wondered? If so, how was it done?

The tournament tai chi that I had encountered and contended with did not seem to offer a satisfactory answer to such an illogical assertion. If that saying was indeed true, it meant that the excesses of physical strength and the use of clever techniques that so frequently led to someone's victory in Push Hands were not "correct" tai chi. I knew all about such inappropriate behaviors from my own experiences in winning and losing matches. It would also mean that, despite my victories, my understanding and practice of tai chi were incorrect as well.

Instead of just competing in more Push Hands events, I wanted to understand for myself if and how "soft overcomes hard". Could the cultivation of "internal energy" actually yield any useful results in the context of Push Hands and applied martial arts? If I'd been declared the winner of these matches and received competitive honors and recognition, how could my path to winning have been the wrong one?

It was not until I first encountered Master Huang, Sheng Shyan that I witnessed an authentic demonstration of this fabled "four ounces" principle in action. Only then did I see the truth of it. His movements that day were so minimal that they were nearly undetectable. Yet, those gentle, imperceptible gestures had a devastating effect on his practice partners. He simply scattered them whenever and wherever he chose. No one was harmed; but, no one was exempt from that outcome. It was a truly baffling thing to watch. His remarkable abilities were the inspiration for my quest to discover how this was done. My efforts to establish a student/teacher relationship with Master Huang are described in Chapter Five.

After years of training and practice with my teachers and from my own experiences, I have since been able to find a practical and sensible solution to that legendary "four ounces" mystery. I found my answer to the question, "How is this done?" Be advised, it is not something easily achieved; but it certainly is accessible to any tai chi student who is willing to do the principle-based work required.

The solution I sought gradually emerged from my lengthy study of tai chi and my related studies in Confucian philosophy, Taoist philosophy, acupuncture, and Traditional Chinese Medicine ("TCM"). This work enabled me to steadily develop, test, and refine my "Seven Principles for Tai Chi Practice". Faithfully pursued, these universal principles make possible the gradual growth, continual accumulation, and successful development of tai chi's remarkable *nei jin*, "internal energy" power.

As a more harmonious alternative to Push Hands, I also created my "Search Center" training method. This "soft way" is equally applicable to both solo practice and dealing with an "opponent" in partner work. It is an effective means for training the proper cultivation and use of "internal energy" power during a paired exercise situation. Through the practice of the various inter-active drills involved, the student's ability to utilize "the soft way" is carefully developed. "Search Center" can be performed in either a "cooperative/collaborative" manner or, preferably only after considerable training and with sufficient experience, in an "uncooperative/competitive" manner.

The training method which I established emphasizes the use of the mind/intent (*Yi*) rather than the use of physical strength and brute force (*Li*) to control an opponent. The training fosters an ever-deepening state of relaxation *(Sung)* during solo form practice. This *Sung* state, in both body and mind, allows the student to recognize and cultivate the resultant "soft power" which gradually emerges. In partner work, he or she then couples the "soft power" with the heightened sense of tactile awareness gained from the slightest sensation of touching one's partner. It is through partner work that tai chi's "listening energy" skills (*ting jin*) are attained. When a well-developed "listening energy" ability is combined with the use of mind/intent (*Yi*), the practitioner can then effectively make use of the "soft power" cultivated during tai chi form practice.

Nevertheless, when confronted with a partner's hard strength and "dull force" the student cannot just counter by thinking about using some ill-defined, "soft way" response. Instead, to be practical, the student must also learn how to yield the physical body and neutralize that incoming force. Indeed, to yield rather than offer resistance is a well-known lesson in all the various styles of tai chi. Yet, yielding the body is only one part of the art. You also need to be able to utilize the internal chi cultivated and contained in "the soft way" as an effective instrument for simultaneously returning that incoming force. This means that you have to know how to use the appropriate tool, at the proper time and place to achieve the desired result. For example, if you compare a golf ball and a table tennis ball side-by-side they are seen to be about the same size. Yet, if you choose the wrong one for the game you are playing, the result will be extremely unsatisfactory. You need to choose the right one for the game you want to play.

Since starting on this tai chi path my ambition has been to constantly improve my understanding of this art and to contribute to its evolution and advancement for the next generation. Having now completed over forty-five years of concentrated study and effort, I want to share what I've learned so that others may benefit from my experience and enjoy long and healthy lives. Sharing this hard-won knowledge with others, particularly the next generation of tai chi students, is my principal reason for writing this book.

My tai chi journey toward finding an answer to the riddle of how "four ounces can move a thousand pounds" began in the following way.

• *A Cultural Tradition of Exercise:* Every Chinese child grows up witnessing the adults going about their daily routine of physical fitness activities. Indeed, my first memory of seeing anyone do tai chi is that of watching my own father's practice. But, being only a child, I took no real interest in any of it.

These days, even if they don't engage in it themselves, everyone understands that regular, daily exercise is an important part of living a healthy life. For a large segment of the Chinese population, exercise is not just thought to be an important part of a healthy life; it is done daily. In Chinese society, such a regimen has an exceedingly long tradition. Each day, wherever in the world there is a sizeable Chinese community, the public parks are notably busy in the early morning hours with people practicing their exercise routines. An astonishing variety of activities is in evidence wherever you look.

Some people will be exercising in groups, some alone. Some will simply be walking briskly. Some will be jogging in the Western manner. One or two will be walking vigorously backward, head turned over their shoulders to see where they are going. Some will be standing completely still for long periods while holding their limbs in a particular position. Others may be seen standing near a large tree, arms spread as if to embrace it. There may even be ballroom dancing with its recorded music spreading into the park's morning air. Among the women, some will be moving gracefully in silent, rhythmic synchronization while waving silk scarves. Other women may flourish colorful fans, certainly the most deceptive of weapons. This they will expertly maneuver in unison, periodically producing its distinctive sound by opening and closing it with a brisk flick of the wrist. The effect of such action is startling and dramatic. Passersby cannot help but look and be delighted.

It is also likely to see people engaged in Chi Kung (Qigong, Qi Gong, Chi Gong) exercises of every type. Chi Kung practice usually involves a combination of movement, meditation, and breathing exercises which are designed to promote health and reduce stress. It is considered to be both a preventive and a curative regimen. There are numerous and diverse Chi Kung exercises. Some consist of dynamic actions while others are less active or even static. Regardless of type, all of them are designed to develop and nurture a person's vital, life-force energy, one's "chi". The term Chi Kung is translated as Chi = breath, gas, air, vapor, and Kung = force or power. Taken together, the two words also imply a sense of accomplishment achieved as a result of prolonged and conscientious practice. In addition to the physical movements, the sequences can also include a variety of mental exercises and visualization techniques. Chi Kung exercises are frequently included in martial arts classes and I often feature them in my tai chi classes.

Among the morning's activities, there will certainly be displays of various complex and sophisticated martial arts routines as well. "Hard styles" and "soft styles" will be demonstrated by men and women of all ages. Park-goers are likely to see empty hand forms and even some traditional weapons such as swords, sabers, and staffs. In addition to the various types of tai chi form practice, there are often groups engaged in the competitive, partner practice known as Push Hands (*Tui Shou*). The martial arts are as much a part of Chinese life as baseball, football or soccer are in Western life. Seeing them being performed in the parks would not be at all surprising to anyone. What would be surprising is not to see them there.

• *A Lifelong Interest in Athletics:* Like many young people, from an early age I had an interest and aptitude for all types of sports activities. However, as a child, I suffered from rather severe asthma. My breathing was frequently labored and difficult. I couldn't run very far without being completely winded and exhausted. This debilitating condition sapped my confidence and made me feel anxious and self-conscious. At the age of twelve, I decided that I could no longer tolerate the limitations that asthma was placing on my life. I felt that I needed to take charge of things and needed to challenge myself to engage in more physical activities. I thought that the increased discipline resulting from a regular practice routine would be good for me both physically and mentally.

Once I'd resolved to redirect my life, deciding which activity to pursue was an easy choice. The sport of gymnastics had always interested me; so, I joined the local team and soon became caught up in the world of men's competitive gymnastics.

The training was rigorous. For example, as part of our practice, we would scale a three-story wall using only a thick rope to aid our "walk" up its side. We would also challenge each other to do a handstand and then climb up and down a staircase while "walking" on our hands, feet extended upward toward the ceiling. To accomplish that, you needed extremely good balance and strong shoulders and arms.

We were expected to participate in all the men's events but my personal favorites were the parallel bars, high bar, and the floor exercise with its many leaps, tumbles, and demonstrations of balance and strength. I immersed myself in practice seven days a week and thrived on the discipline and hard work required in perfecting my routines.

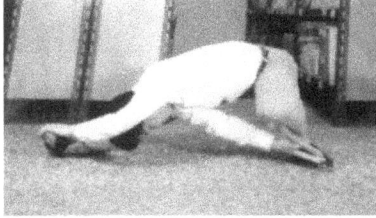

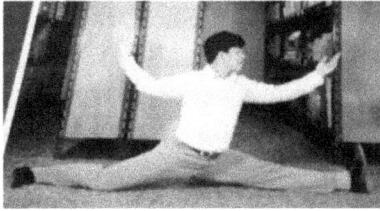

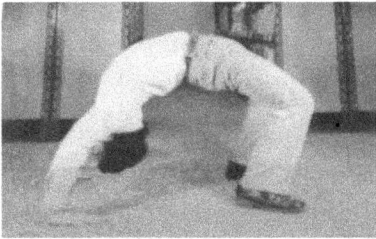

Henry Wang, Gymnast

While still a teenager I was also drawn to the martial arts. At that time Lee Jun-fan, better known as Bruce Lee (1940-1973), had become a world-renowned martial artist and a Chinese-American movie star. He was born in San Francisco, California but was raised and lived in Hong Kong until his late teens. His father was also a famous Chinese actor and Bruce had been in many movies while he lived in Hong Kong. He also appeared as "Kato" in the United States television show "The Green Hornet" in 1966-1967. In addition to his acting career, Bruce had founded the hybrid martial art system he called "Jeet Kune Do". He developed it as an outgrowth from Wing Chun, another well-known and well-regarded style of Chinese martial art.

Many young men in Taiwan, and probably everywhere there was a movie screen, wanted to be like Bruce. With his example to inspire me, I started my own martial arts studies in 1967. At age sixteen, I began to study judo and the hardstyle Shaolin arts in Taipei where my family lived. As my interest in martial arts grew more and more serious my participation in gymnastics began to gradually decrease. Finally, I simply shifted my focus entirely to martial arts and completely gave up gymnastics. I continued my martial arts training until I was required to enter the army a few years later.

• *Army Service:* In the early 1970s military service was compulsory for all, able-bodied men born in Taiwan. At that time, two years of active duty in the Republic of China's (Taiwanese) armed forces were required of us. So, in 1971, when I was 20 years old, I became a soldier. I was assigned to the army's largest branch, the infantry. One of the good things about being in the infantry was that it allowed me to continue to pursue my interest in martial arts.

For hand-to-hand combat training, the army taught a combination of gung fu (hardstyle fighting) and Taekwondo, the formidable Korean martial art known for its powerful kicking techniques. The military instructors I encountered were exceptionally competent and they delighted in perfecting their techniques on each group of incoming recruits. They regularly and methodically put us to the test and seemed to become more skillful each day. There were some days when I found them to be a little too enthusiastic about their work and my aching body agreed. Nevertheless, I was keen to learn all that I could so I did not mind the rigorous training. I thoroughly enjoyed it most of the time.

Building on my existing skills and under the watchful eyes of my instructors, over the next several months I gained additional competence and proficiency in combat-type fighting. My progress was such that I soon left the ranks of being a pupil and found myself assigned as a martial arts instructor as part of my military duties. That assignment was my initial exposure to the challenges and rewards of being a martial arts teacher. As both a combatant and trainer, the experience I gained was to be of considerable value to me in the following years.

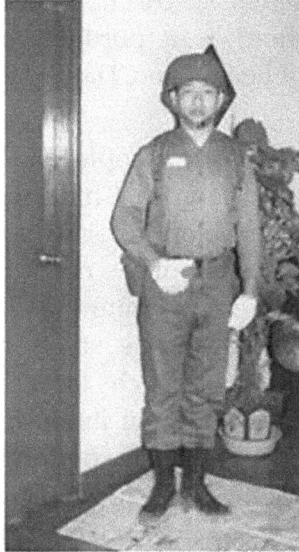

Master Wang, age 20. Full army dress.

Some young men are meant to be career soldiers but that way of life was not the correct way for me. When my two-year commitment ended, I left the service and returned to civilian life where I entered college to study journalism. It was then that I also began my study of tai chi. Moreover, that was also the year I first met my future wife, Ivy. As it happened, 1973 was a watershed year in my life.

• *My First Tai Chi Teacher:* Like most people, I suppose that I was initially attracted to tai chi for a variety of reasons. It was graceful and serene to watch yet had the paradoxical reputation of being a highly practical and effective method of self-defense. It also was understood to have many health-giving and health-sustaining properties. But, in addition to all those things, I was particularly interested in tai chi's supposed ability to soften one's temper. My time in the army led me to develop a rather quick temper and this was a trait that I wanted to subdue.

The Kwun Lun Pai style, an old and well-regarded style from mainland China, was the very first style of tai chi that I learned. The teacher came from my father's mainland home province of Hubei and had taught my father tai chi many years before he taught me. Hubei (a/k/a Yangzhou) is a northern province of China that surrounds the cities of Beijing and Tianjin. Its name means "north of the Yellow River".

Historically, the Chinese people have largely lived a rural, agrarian life. It was common in China for an individual village, region, or province to develop a particularly local style of martial arts. This was a consequence of the need to provide for their own, local security against common criminals. Of course, there are many similarities among these various styles but there is also great diversity. Kwun Lun Pai is one such "local style" and is not very well known outside of China. Many of its postures are similar to those done by Shaolin boxers but they are performed more slowly.

• *My Other Tai Chi Studies:* Next, I also studied the 108 posture Yang Style long form. Later still, I learned the 37 posture short form which Professor Cheng, Man-ch'ing developed as an abbreviated version of the Yang Style long form.

In my classes, I continue to use the postures and sequence of Professor Cheng's form as the basis for instruction. However, we do not perform them in precisely the same manner in which I was originally taught. The majority of the shapes and the sequence of postures generally remain the same and would thus be familiar to the numerous students worldwide who have studied the Professor's form. However, there are many differences in both emphasis and execution. For example, I have my students learn to do the entire sequence of postures from both the right side and left side of the body. This was never done in the Professor's classes and he actively discouraged it. Also, in executing some segments (e.g., brush knee to the low punch) my students step backward rather than forward when stringing the movements together. They are also asked and expected to conduct all their tai chi activities, both solo form and "Search Center" partner practice, in harmony with my Seven Principles. Nevertheless, the Professor's well-designed routine provides the most useful template for their practice.

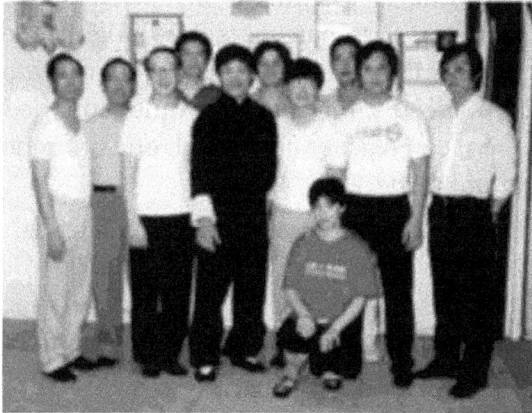

Students in one of Master Wang's tai chi classes in Taiwan.
Master Wang, black uniform.

• *The Influence of Four Exceptional Teachers*: When I began my study of tai chi, most Chinese tai chi masters still took a very traditional approach in their teaching methods. One of the first things a prospective student was expected to do was to build a relationship with the teacher. The purpose of this "getting to know you" phase was to demonstrate to the teacher the depths of the student's desire to learn the art.

Traditionally, the master/student, teacher/pupil relationship in any discipline has been highly regarded in Chinese society and accorded great respect. That relationship also carried with it a series of reciprocal duties owed between the two parties; duties which were taken quite seriously. Consequently, the teacher of any martial art wanted to have confidence in the student's sincerity of interest before undertaking the obligations associated with such instruction. He needed at least some assurance that he would not be wasting time on an irresponsible, undependable, or unworthy pupil.

Once this initial test of character had been passed, the master would agree to accept the student and perhaps, later still, would make the student part of his "indoor" group. Certain "hidden" portions of a particular family's martial art would customarily only be revealed to "indoor" students within the family's bloodline. Occasionally, a few, fortunate outsiders might be deemed worthy enough to be admitted into the privileged "indoor" group. This "indoor" acceptance by the master would often lead to a life-long relationship between teacher and pupil, one of friendship, devotion, trust, and mutual respect.

In my tai chi career, it has been such friendship, offered and returned, which has meant all the difference to my development as a martial artist. It has enabled me to connect with many different and talented people and have exposure to many different ideas about tai chi. The instruction and friendship of four men, in particular, showed me the way. These men were the most influential in my advancement as a martial artist. Arranged in the order in which I met them they are: (1) the general, Master Yang, Yu Zhen, (2) the professor of philosophy, Master Zheng, Yang Ming (3) the I-Chuan expert, Master Do, Tsu Jang, and (4) Master Huang, Sheng Shyan, the Malaysian personification and exemplar of the soft way.

◆ ◆ ◆

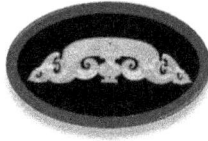

Chapter 2: The General

AFTER OUR MARRIAGE in 1974, Ivy and I moved from the capital city, Taipei, to the nearby district in the southern part of Taipei county called Xindian (Sindian). Although it is full of apartment buildings serving those working in the capital, it is an area of considerable natural beauty since it is located near the northern end of Taiwan's Central Mountain Range. A dam was built on a local river which created the well-known Bitan Lake (Green Lake).

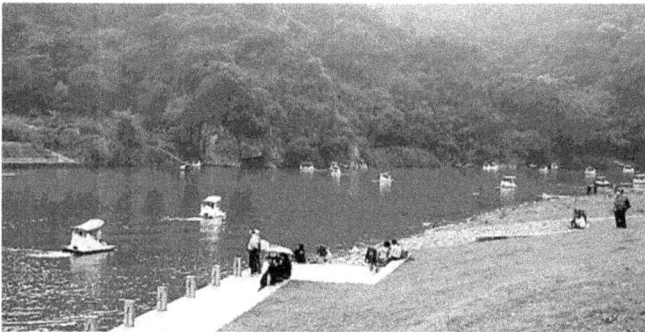

Bitan Lake

The surrounding steep, green cliffs and the lake's blue-green water make it a favorite scenic destination, particularly on weekends. The area has many good hiking trails due to its proximity to the mountains. The local market and the lakeside teahouses are also a big draw and certainly worth a visit. Typical Taiwanese dishes can easily be found in the restaurants near the lake.

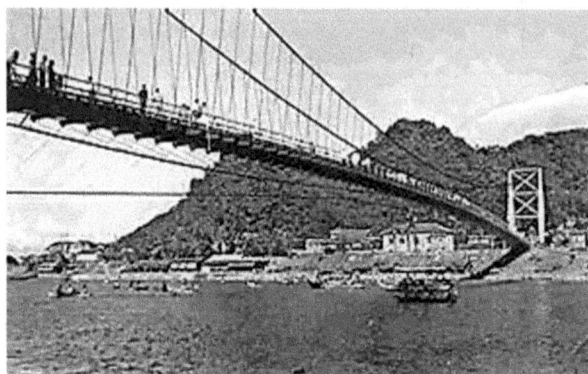

Pedestrian Suspension Bridge, Bitan Lake

• *The Yang Style Long Form:* To broaden my martial arts knowledge and see what further use could be made of my army training, I decided that I should learn more about tai chi. Tai chi was of particular interest because it had the paradoxical reputation of being both a means for cultivating good health and, at the same time, it was known as a powerful method of self-defense. After we'd settled in, I decided to go to the local park to look for a teacher. Martial arts of all types, including tai chi, are often taught in the public parks so I thought that it was likely that I could find a class there. This meant that I would have to get up much earlier and head to the park before going to work.

According to traditional Chinese medicine ("TCM"), the energy contained in our body's various organ systems continuously cycles through those organs in two-hour segments each day. In related Taoist thought, the early morning hours, particularly between 5:00 a.m. and 7:00 a.m., are considered the best time to practice tai chi and other forms of exercise. By adopting an early-morning schedule, we can obtain the full advantage of this periodic cycle and maximize the health benefits obtainable during any twenty-four-hour period.

As a practical matter, given Taiwan's tropical climate and high humidity, the early morning is also the most enjoyable time for physical exertion of any sort. With this in mind, I made a point of getting to the park promptly at the start of the day.

16

I soon found and introduced myself to Master Tzou who taught the Yang Style Long Form (108 postures). His group met each morning at 6:30 a.m. Both men and women attended the classes. The turnout varied each day but usually, the women outnumbered the men. This is not at all unusual for classes held in a park setting. I was one of the younger members of the group. Most of the other attendees were middle-aged or older. Some were retirees.

There were no verbal instructions during Master Tzou's practice sessions. The students were expected to just follow along and copy the pattern and sequence of movements performed by their teacher. Learning was done purely by observing and doing. This is a time-honored, traditional method of teaching martial arts in Chinese society and I was quite comfortable with this approach. Of course, my previous years of martial arts practice made it that much easier for me to familiarize myself with and perform the material being presented. Reasonably soon, I was able to learn the entire sequence of postures and began to include the Long Form in my daily practice routine.

• *Meeting the General:* My father's family lineage was originally from Hubei province in mainland China. As a result of my subsequent participation in various Push Hands competitions, I was destined to meet another Hubei native who had an important influence on my tai chi practice. In 1975 a mutual acquaintance from Hubei introduced me to Master Yang, Yu-Jen. Master Yang was a retired general in the Taiwanese army. Like many others, Master Yang had relocated from mainland China to Taiwan in 1949. He was not a student of Cheng Man-ch'ing. Instead, he had studied North Tao Tai Chi and also a different style taught by Master Wang, Yen-nien. A short while later I was fortunate to also study Push Hands with Master Wang, Yen-nien's group.

When I met him, Master Yang, Yu-Jen was the Secretary of the National Tai Chi Chuan Association of Taiwan. He later became its President. At that time, he was traveling around the country to promote the growth of the association which had only recently been founded. Again, good fortune and the Chinese "social networking" custom of *"guanxi"* had served me well.

As Secretary of the association, Master Yang had access to the group's entire library of tai chi books. He graciously loaned many of them to me and I studied them closely, page by page. These books were a tremendous resource and provided me with many hours of informative and pleasurable reading. He and I would have many long conversations about their contents. We would discuss the various ideas different authors had about tai chi, its underlying premises, and its philosophy. I came to better understand that tai chi was not only for improving one's health; it was also an effective method of self-defense. This martial aspect of tai chi was particularly interesting to me because of my army background in Taekwondo and my skills in teaching combat fighting.

A few weeks after we first met, I brought him a particularly troublesome question with which I'd become preoccupied. I was curious to learn just how tai chi made use of yielding and the "soft way" to build a skillful method of self-defense. Such an approach to martial arts was contrary to everything that I had been taught and everything that I had been doing up until then. While I was skeptical about its usefulness in an actual fight, the contrary nature of this approach to self-defense intrigued me. I had to see for myself if what I'd been reading was fact or fiction so I politely asked Master Yang to teach me how this was done. He graciously agreed to do so.

At that time, the National Tai Chi Chuan Association had only one meeting room and there was no suitable space to practice there. Master Yang was kind enough to invite me to his home for lessons and practice. Each weekend I would go to his house in a nearby town for a training session. Master Yang's style of tai chi was called "Jin-sun-pie" (Quin-lun-pie). I followed his movements carefully and practiced his style to the best of my abilities. Sometimes after practice, we would go to lunch and eat steamed buns which were items he particularly liked. Our weekly lessons soon resulted in the development of a strong and lasting friendship. He had a long life and died at the age of 103.

• *Yang Family Style Push Hands Practice:* Once I had finished learning the postures and sequence of that particular form, Master Yang told me about a Push Hands group that met every Sunday outside Taipei. They got together at a two-story building in a suburban district. There was a business on the first floor and the second floor was the Push Hands classroom.

Master Yang took me there and introduced me to the group's teacher, Master Wang Yen-nien (1914-2008). He was a 4th generation teacher of Yangjia Michuan Taijiquan (Yang Family Secret Taijiquan). Before moving to Taiwan in 1949, Master Wang had learned that style's full system from Zhang Qinlin (1888-1967), a 3rd generation teacher who had himself studied under both Yang Jianhou and Yang's son, Yang Chengfu. I later learned that Master Wang Yen-nien and Professor Cheng Man-ch'ing both had the same teacher. Not Yang Chang Fu but someone else. I'm not sure who that person was.

In Master Wang Yen-nien's group, the Push Hands instruction included both fixed-step and moving-step routines. Although tai chi is commonly described as one of the "soft styles" of martial arts, the Push Hands that went on in that upstairs classroom was most definitely not soft practice. Tatami mats had been hung from the walls and the losing player was forcibly hurled into them. Throughout a training session, the room was filled with the constant sound of bodies repeatedly thudding against those solid barriers. Every successful push was usually followed by a resultant grunt or groan from the unfortunate recipient. I was thankful for the protection provided by those mats, even though it was undeniably limited. The solid impact produced by a "good push" could largely eliminate their meager and inadequate cushioning effect. On such occasions, one's back collided with the wall as if there were no padding at all.

Despite the many times that I was thrown against those classroom walls, I enjoyed the training challenges presented by this "friendly assault" type of practice. Fortunately, my army background had equipped me with some effective martial arts skills; so, I was often able to catch my opponent's "hard point" and push them out. A "hard point" is a place on the body or positioning of the body in which a person becomes momentarily immobilized or "stuck". It renders the person unable to respond in a timely and appropriate way to counter the partner's attack; as a result, they become vulnerable. On those occasions, it was my partner's body bouncing off the wall and not my own. How satisfying that was! Of course, I did not always "win" but I thrived on the spirited competition.

• *My First Tai Chi Tournament:* At one point during those years, the National Tai Chi Chuan Association wanted to promote tai chi by holding its very first tai chi Push Hands tournament. This was in 1976 I believe. Each of the various tai chi groups around the country was invited to send a representative. I was asked to compete. So, I went as a representative of my hometown, Xindian (Sindian).

There were about twenty different tai chi groups in the association. For the tournament, they were divided into three sectors: a north island group, a south island group, and a central island group. It was decided that the contestants from each group would compete among themselves and there would be three tournament champions, one from each group. There was to be no division of contestants by weight class or age groups or years of training, etc. The tournament was truly "open".

The many hours of Push Hands practice with Master Wang Yen-nien's students along with my army experiences made me confident that I had the skills which might enable me to do well and perhaps even win in my group. Indeed, I did win my matches and thus became champion of the north island group.

At that time my tai chi still used lots of strength. While my use of muscle and what I would now consider "dull force" had helped me win, my body paid the price. When the tournament ended, I had aches and pains everywhere. After that victory, it took me a full week to recover.

In retrospect, that tournament provided no evidence or examples whatsoever of tai chi's famous maxim that "four ounces can move one thousand pounds". Quite to the contrary, it had been a rough, forceful, physical event. I left the tournament pleased that I had won but thinking that maybe this famous tai chi expression was simply empty words and not actually true. My soft skills had not yet been developed. I still had much muscular force to give up and a long way to go in that regard. It wasn't until a few years later that I both witnessed and was on the receiving end of the truth of that classic "four ounces" saying. It was still even longer before I was able to embody the expression of that truth myself. (See Chapter Five, "The Malaysian Master".)

• *My Next Teacher:* Many of the social and business relationships in Chinese culture, both in Taiwan and in mainland China, are initiated and revolve around the customary practice known as "*guanxi*". Although considerably more nuanced and sophisticated, the notion behind "*guanxi*" might be summarized as "It's not what you know; it's who you know". It is a refined method of personal "social networking" and relationship building via "connections". This significant and influential system is based on a reciprocal exchange of favors and introductions. There are similar "networking" systems in many other cultures around the world. When considering the path which one's life may take, the importance of karma coupled with a well-placed and well-timed introduction cannot be overstated. My relationship with Master Yang led me to my next tai chi teacher. It was "*guanxi*" that opened the door.

Master Wang Yen-nien was then Chairman of the Tai Chi Association when Master Yang presented me for an introduction. (Master Yang was later to become Chairman himself.) Master Wang Yen-nien was a practitioner of another tai chi form known as North Jin Sun tai chi.

The movements of this particular form were quite different from those of the Cheng Man-ch'ing form. For example, in the Cheng Man-ch'ing style, considerable emphasis was placed on maintaining an even height of the pelvis/waist throughout the form. In the North Jin Sun style, the emphasis was exactly the opposite; there was a considerable change in height, both up and down, throughout the form. Many other details of the North Jin Sun style were entirely different from the Cheng Man-ch'ing form which I had come to know. Once again, these stylistic differences caused me some concern and I wondered whether I could ever reconcile all the various lessons I was learning.

◆ ◆ ◆

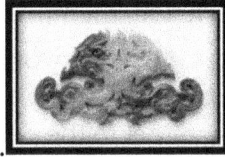

Chapter 3: The Philosopher & His Friends

THE COMMUTE TO work each day from my house in Xindian (Sindian) to Taipei would take me about forty-five minutes each way on my bicycle. In the evenings, before returning home, I would stop at the playground of a local high school to practice my tai chi form.

One day I noticed that an older gentleman had stopped to watch me practice. Surprisingly, he then stayed on until I'd completed an entire round of form. This was rather unusual and certainly unexpected. Most passers-by would not have paid any attention to me. In Chinese society, a lone person practicing martial arts was a familiar and ordinary sight. If any passing pedestrian bothered to pause at all it might be only for a minute or two at most. It was uncommon for anyone to linger for the entire ten minutes or so that it takes to complete an entire round of form. I wondered why he was so interested. Afterward, he came over and started a conversation.

"What style of tai chi is that?", he asked.

"(Quin Lun) Jin sun pie style."

"The way you move is not the proper way to do tai chi.", he said.

"What do you mean?", I asked.

"Have you ever heard of Professor Cheng Man-ch'ing?"

"I've heard of him. I know he was a famous tai chi teacher but I've never seen him."

"I was a student of Professor Cheng Man-ch'ing. I have been doing tai chi for twenty years. Each evening I walk to this school. If you are interested, I can teach you the tai chi style I learned from the Professor."

We talked some more. I was very open to the idea of learning tai chi from a variety of sources. I wanted as much exposure as I could get to the perspective others had to offer about this elusive art. It impressed me that he had been taught by Professor Cheng who was a man of considerable reputation and skills. Additionally, the fact that this elderly stranger had been doing tai chi for such a long time also indicated that he took it seriously. I thought he must be pretty good so I immediately agreed. This was how I met the philosophy professor, Master Zheng, Yang Ming.

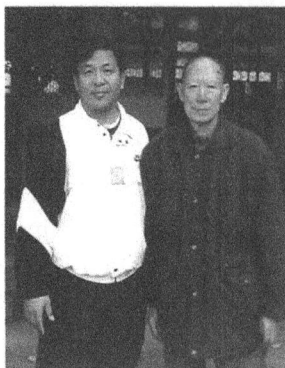

Master Zheng, Yang Ming
Henry Wang, left

From then on, each evening that I came to the schoolyard, he gave me a new posture to learn. I wasn't a traditional "formal" student of Master Zheng. He later had other students as well.

Master Zheng is a very polite person. Before teaching philosophy at the university, he had been a general in the army intelligence service and fought against the Japanese in World War II. When he retired from the army, he remained in government service doing civilian work in another government office.

One day he invited me to his home. In his living room, there was an autographed picture from Chiang Kai-shek, the former president of the Republic of China, Taiwan. There was also an original painting done by Professor Cheng Man-ch'ing. In addition to his skills as a martial artist, Professor Cheng has been described as a "Master of Five Excellences": painting, poetry, calligraphy, traditional Chinese medicine, and tai chi chuan.

I studied with Master Zheng for about ten years until I left Taiwan and moved to Canada. Beyond its being a challenging physical discipline, one of the appealing aspects of tai chi is that it also encourages the development of friendships as part of its underlying philosophy. One of my most satisfying tai chi experiences has been the friendship that Master Zheng and I developed over those years.

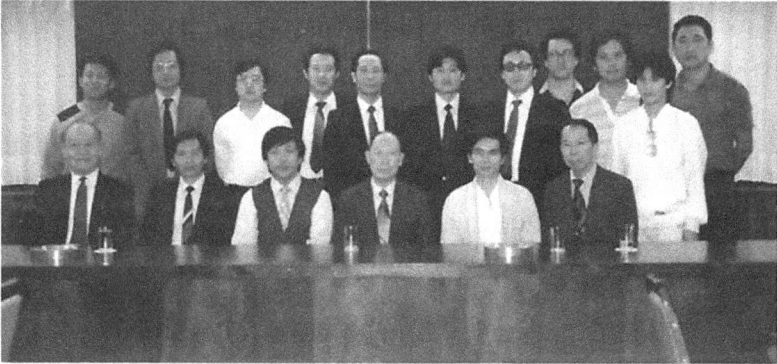

Tai Chi Study Group.
Seated: Master Zheng center, Henry Wang, third from left.

• *Tai Chi Practice with Master Zheng:* Master Zheng had already retired from his teaching position as a professor of philosophy at the Wu Taipei University when I met him. He did not have a bricks-and-mortar tai chi school. Instead, he and his small group of students met just once a week on Sundays in Xindian (Sindian). He named his school "Chur Lo Suh" or "Extremely Soft School". Primarily because we were constantly practicing Push Hands (*Tui Shou*) and people were interested in that, the number of students gradually increased. However, as is common in the martial arts, people tended to come and go and the group never exceeded ten people at any one time.

When I met him, Master Zheng was over seventy years old and the Push Hands he did was extremely effective. I was a much younger man and, having been a former hand-to-hand combat instructor, I expected to be able to move him without much trouble. Imagine my surprise when I could not. This "old man" had a tremendous root and, despite my army skills and advantage in years, I found it very difficult to move him.

He would constantly tell me that I was too hard. He emphasized that all aspects of tai chi movements, including Push Hands, should be soft like water. Soft, like Lao Tse's philosophy. I must admit that I was somewhat skeptical of this advice since I found that his body was not as soft and pliable as he insisted that I should become. Nevertheless, he certainly had a good root and I was very pleased and fortunate to learn from and practice with someone who had such considerable skills.

• *The Tao and Tai Chi:* Tai chi is not just a physical exercise. It is an art whose principles are also deeply embedded in Chinese philosophy and culture, particularly the Taoist philosophy of Lao Tse. Although he never mentioned it at our first meeting, Master Zheng, was a famous philosophy professor in Taiwan. In addition to his other scholarly work, Master Zheng had a special interest in Taoist philosophy and had written three, well-regarded books on the teachings of Lao Tse. The books explained how Lao Tse's philosophy related to the world of art, to the Taoist religion, and to chi itself. It is unfortunate that as yet none of his writings are available in English.

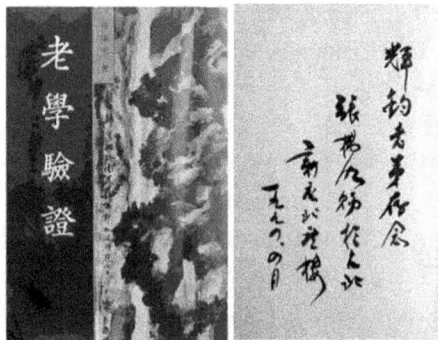

Book re Study of Lao Tse
Master Zheng's Gift to Henry Wang, April 1994

The Tao Te Ching, the principal philosophical work attributed to Lao Tse, has only about five thousand Chinese characters. Although it is not very long, it is difficult to understand. Master Zheng explained and clarified its substance and essential teachings to me over the many years I studied with him. Each Sunday, after our tai chi practice, he would present one or two sentences from Lao Tse's teaching and we would discuss their meaning and significance.

During this time, I also was able to attend many of the lectures and speeches he still gave at the university after his retirement. He was the one person who helped me to understand the relationship between the philosophy of Lao Tse and its applicability to the principles underlying the postures and patterns of movement found in the art of tai chi.

For example, the Taoists place considerable emphasis on humankind's place in and relationship to nature and the natural world. They maintain that the doing of any action should not be forced and should not use force. Instead, it should be allowed to unfold according to its nature and in its own time. The actions and movements of tai chi are directly related to this idea of following nature's way.

• *Being a Colleague of Cheng Man-ch'ing:* I learned that it was through their mutual interest in philosophy that Master Zheng had first met and became friends with Professor Cheng, Man-ch'ing. This occurred when they both lived in mainland China. Before meeting Professor Cheng, he had already studied tai chi with other teachers. Soon after they met, he began to study tai chi with Professor Cheng as well.

He told me that Professor Cheng's tai chi was extremely soft. As a result, the Professor had developed such a high degree of "listening energy" (*ting jin*) that he was able to detect very early what the opponent intended to do. Knowing that intention enabled him to neutralize his adversary's actions and allowed the Professor to readily turn the tables on him.

• *A Pupil in Common with Professor Cheng:* At one point, Master Zheng told me that he was also one of Benjamin Lo's (Lo, Pang Jeng) (1927-2018) philosophy teachers. The many people in Taiwan, Canada, the United States, and Europe who practice the Cheng Man-ch'ing style knew and highly respected Master Lo and his abilities. Master Lo was Professor Cheng's patient and first pupil when the

Professor moved to Taiwan in 1949. For a time, he lived in Professor Cheng's household and was perhaps his last "indoor" student. He studied with Cheng for twenty-six years, until Cheng's death in 1975.

Master Lo emigrated to San Francisco, California in 1974 where he founded the Universal Tai Chi Chuan Association and taught tai chi for many, many years. He also traveled extensively throughout the world giving workshops and seminars. He worked tirelessly to preserve and pass on the Professor's lessons and he expected his students to work hard as well.

• *The Cheng Man-ch'ing Group:* As I've mentioned, early in my tai chi career I joined in various tai chi Push Hands competitions. At one point, I joined a tai chi tournament sponsored by the National Tai Chi Chuan Association. A reporter from a local television station put my match on the television news. It was after I had joined that particular tai chi competition that Master Zheng introduced me to various other teachers from the Cheng, Man-ch'ing school, and its lineage.

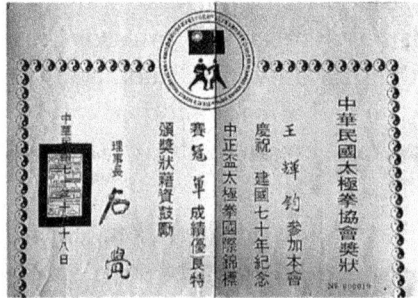

Certificate for the Gold Medal Awarded to Master Wang
The National Tai Chi Chuan Association of the Republic of China
October 18, 1981

Master Zheng was friends with many people in the various Cheng, Man-ch'ing groups in Taiwan. After we had practiced for several months, Master Zheng said he felt that I was making progress and getting better in my tai chi form and Push Hands. He offered to introduce me to a couple of other Cheng, Man-ch'ing tai chi groups which were led by two men who had also been direct students of Professor Cheng.

Once again *"guanxi"* had helped open tai chi doors for me. As a result of my introduction through Master Zheng, I was able to attend practice sessions at Professor, Cheng, Man-ch'ing's Shr Jung School in Taipei. At that time, the leader of the group with Master Liu, Shih Hung (Liu, Xiheng) (1915-2009) who was the Professor's first disciple in Taiwan. His students practiced at Tai Dah University.

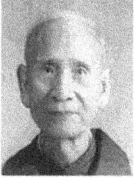

Liu, Shih Hung

Thereafter, I would regularly attend their practices and have many friends and associates at that school to this day. I frequently see them when I travel to Taiwan to visit my relatives.

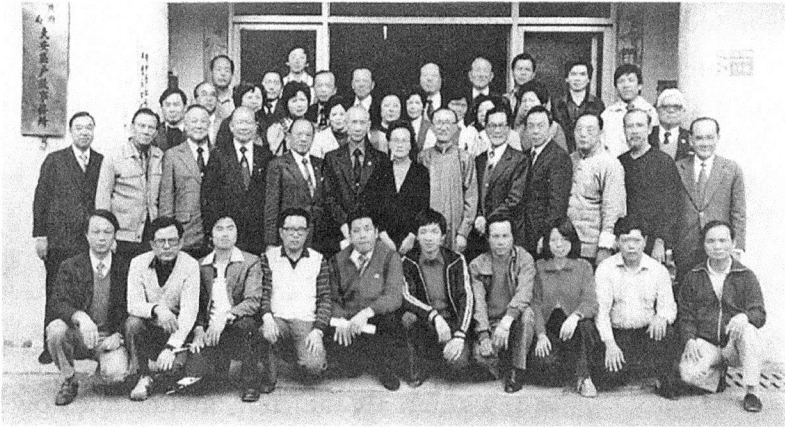

Cheng Man Ching Group, Taipei, Taiwan. (c. 1976)
Master Liu, Shih Hung, second row, 6th from left.
Henry Wang, top row, right side end.

In addition to meeting Master Liu, I was also able to meet Master Gunn, Sheeow Tzo. Master Gunn was also a student of Cheng Man-ch'ing but he was junior to Master Liu in that regard. Again, it was *"guanxi"* which paved the way for my entrée into the classes conducted by Master Gunn. As I've mentioned, the philosophy professor, Master Zheng, Yang Ming had been a high-ranking general in the nationalist army. Master Gunn, who had also been an officer in the army, had met and worked with Master Zheng while both were in the military. Through this connection and the gracious intercession of Master Zheng, I was readily accepted into the group and quickly became very close to Master Gunn.

As a result of these two introductions, I had many more chances to practice Push Hands with a variety of very capable players. My competitive skills improved and I didn't feel as many aches and pains after practice. As my skills increased, I continually tried to relate them to the Taoist way. I hoped to better understand how to connect the practical and the philosophical. I wanted my actions to reflect the practical aspects of tai chi as an effective method of self-defense. At the same time, I also wanted my actions to have resulted from following the soft way, the natural way advocated and celebrated in Taoist philosophy.

I considered myself fortunate to be able to study with these highly regarded practitioners. However, I found myself confused by each man's tai chi form because, as far as I was able to observe, they were quite different from each other. Master Liu's steps while doing the form were bigger than Master Gunn's steps. Also, Master Liu's form was executed smoothly whereas the movements of Master Gunn's form were somewhat tighter. I could not understand how two students of the same teacher could end up with tai chi forms that looked so different. Perhaps the explanation was simply that Master Liu was an early student of Cheng Man-ch'ing whereas Master Gunn was a later student.

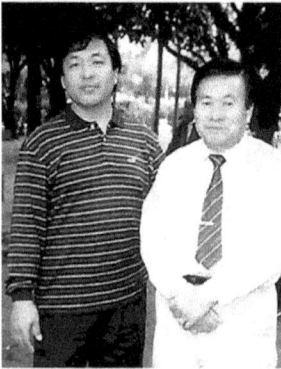

Master Gunn, Sheeow Tzo Henry Wang, left.

The disparity in the styles of these two talented teachers gave me something more to think about. I wondered what the "standard size" of the tai chi form might be. I sought to discover if there was an underlying principle or rule which could reconcile the two contrasting examples these two men presented.

• *Another Influential Teacher:* In April of 2009, I received in the mail an unexpected package from Taiwan. It contained a large book, written in Chinese, which was about the Cheng Man-ch'ing museum that had recently been established in Taipei. The book was a gift from another inspirational teacher and friend, Master Hsu, Yee-Chung, the museum's director. Master Hsu helped establish the museum and had a principal role in getting the whole project going. He raised a large portion of the money needed to acquire the building and fund the construction and exhibition of the museum's collection.

I first met Master Hsu in 1976 at my first competitive Push Hands tournament in Taiwan. I was twenty-five years old. He was a well-regarded journalist and newspaper editor and another of the accomplished teachers from the Cheng Man-ch'ing lineage. When I was privileged to study with him, he was the youngest teacher among that group. I was in my mid-twenties then and all of my teachers were at least forty years older than I was.

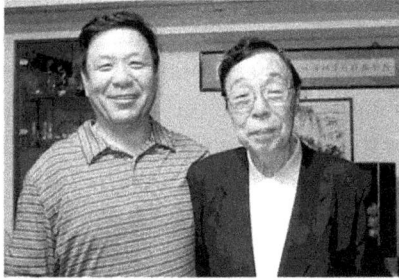

Henry Wang and Master Hsu, Yee-Chung
Taipei, April 2009

Master Hsu's tai chi was quite accomplished and very soft. He continuously encouraged me to develop a stronger root and to relax more. He maintained that relaxation was extremely important if one wanted to obtain a high level of tai chi skills.

Master Hsu has always spoken very highly of his teacher, Professor Cheng. He is quick to point out how very talented the Professor was in many different areas besides martial arts and what a positive influence he had been in Master Hsu's own life.

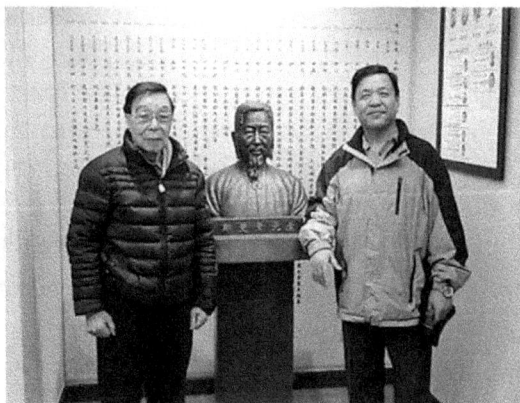

Master Hsu, Yee-Chung and Master Wang
Shr Jung School, Taipei - March 2017

Master Hsu has been the principal successor and leader of the Shr-Jung School which was originally established by Cheng Man-ch'ing in Taiwan. When the Professor moved to New York City in 1964 and established his first tai chi training center there he also called that school the Shr-Jung Center for the Cultural Arts. He used that name yet again in 1973 when he moved the Shr-Jung Tai Center, to its second location in New York City.

Master Hsu has a wonderfully welcoming and friendly personality. Although he was one of my teachers, our relationship was not the rigid and formal master/student one that was so often characteristic of the Chinese martial arts world. It was more on the level of mutual friendship. Master Hsu's kindly and compassionate example was a tremendously positive influence on the development of my teaching style. The friendship and warmth he demonstrated toward me as his student became the model for my interactions with my students.

◆ ◆ ◆

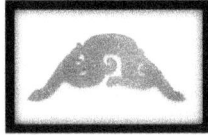

Chapter 4: The I-Chuan Master

ANOTHER OF MY early teachers was Master Do, Tsu Jang. Like Master Zheng, I also met him on the playground of the local high school in Xiandian (Sindian) where I practiced my tai chi form. Master Do would often bring his granddaughter to the playground. While she played with her friends, he would watch me doing tai chi. One day he came over to talk to me.

Master Do was another former military man. Like so many others who did not want to live under Communist rule, he had moved with the nationalist forces to Taiwan in 1949. He had a distinguished career of over thirty years in the air force. Among other things, his duties included teaching sports and fitness training. Coincidentally, fitness training was the type of work I'd chosen to do; so, from the outset, he and I had that in common. He had also studied Western-style boxing and was proficient enough at that type of fighting to win an air force championship.

• *"Yong Yi, Bu Yong Li"*: Master Do was the tai chi teacher who introduced me to the simple-sounding yet puzzling saying *"Yong Yi, Bu Yong Li"* ("Use the Mind, Not Force."). The following years have confirmed this to be an absolutely essential lesson for the attainment of a truly high-level proficiency in one's tai chi practice. I am truly appreciative of his insights in this regard.

The "*Yi*" in the phrase indicates the control and use of the body's "internal chi" energy via conscious control of the mind/intent. In the martial arts context, this use of the "internal chi" is referred to as "neijing" or "neigong" and is contrasted with the use of external force. The "Li" in the phrase refers to the use of the external physical force available from the exertion of muscular strength and strong bones, speed, and timing. "Yong" means "use" and "Bu Yong" means "don't use".

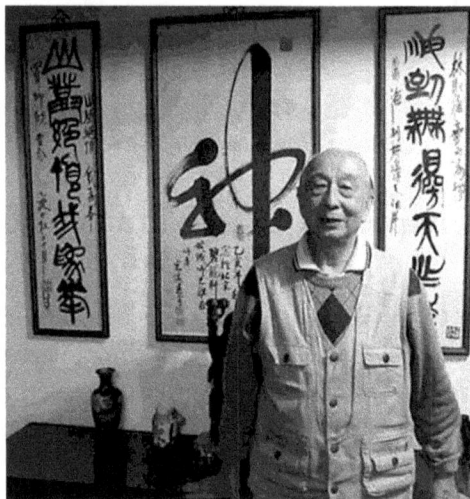

Master·Do,·Tsu·Jang,¶
Taipei··April·2009¶

The deeper lessons which underlie this saying involve understanding, training, and utilizing the Yin/Yang relationship between the body and the mind. This is done by using one's mind and intent to accumulate, strengthen and circulate one's internal energy (the "neijing chi") throughout the entire body; and, the simultaneous ability to direct the manifestation of this "neijing chi" to any single point on our body at will. This is not just a simple mental exercise in "visualization", such as a mere picturing or imagining of such a thing occurring. It is the cultivation and training of an actual, internal physical state. One which is qualitatively different from that occurring in an untrained person who is seen to be making identical external movements and postures. In this context, the body must remain "Sung" (deeply relaxed and free of tension) and soft (Yin) while the engaged mind remains unwaveringly focused and on task (Yang). The training seeks to develop the ability to match the two energies of body and mind, the Yin and Yang, so that the soft, "open" and relaxed body combines naturally with the focused mind and thereby allows the *"neijing chi"* to flow unobstructed to wherever the mind sends it.

I did not truly understand what he meant when he first introduced that concept. Nor did I grasp its true depth and significance. It would take many more years of tai chi study before I was able to utilize that instruction in an applied, practical way against another tai chi player. Only then did I genuinely and fully appreciate the elegance and the true worth of this simple-sounding yet essential lesson. It is this mutual training of mind and body that I have developed in my "Search Center" method's partner work exercises. (See Chapter 13, "Search Center".)

• *No Background in Tai Chi:* I was surprised when I learned that Master Do had never studied tai chi. As a martial artist, he was a devotee of I-Chuan (*Yi Quan*), which is another internal martial arts system. He had studied and practiced it enthusiastically while living in Beijing. However, other demands in his life had necessitated that he put aside his I-Chuan practice for twenty years before being able to resume it.

I had never heard of I-Chuan until I met him. It was not then widely seen in Taiwan and so was still a rather obscure art. I was very curious about what was involved and how it was done.

• *The "Internal Style" Trio:* Hsing-I Chuan, Bagua (Baguazhang, Bāguà Zhǎng), and Tai Chi Chuan (Taijiquan) are certainly the three most commonly known and widely practiced types of the Chinese "internal style" martial arts. Tai chi of course is the one that is most prominent and popular in the West. For those who may be unfamiliar with one or more of them, numerous videos and descriptions of all these arts are readily available on the internet. What follows is a brief and rather simplistic introduction and comparison.

Of the three styles, Hsing-I Chuan is perhaps the most martial in its outward appearance. Hsing-I's powerful movements, often delivered from short distances, are designed to simultaneously defend and attack an adversary. A direct, straight ahead, more linear pattern of actions and footwork are used to invade and occupy the opponent's space. It uses mind/intent, a unified body, and tightly spiraled internal energy in the performance of its angular-looking postures and applications. Even when retreating on a straight line, the Hsing-I practitioner's goal is to regroup and continue a forward offensive whenever possible.

By way of contrast, in Bagua (Baguazhang, Bāguà Zhǎng) the footwork and pattern of movement are circular, not linear. Using distinctive footwork and a limited number of simple-looking yet sophisticated hand changes, the Bagua player walks and moves around the circumference of a circle. While "walking/turning the circle", the upper body faces somewhat inward with the arms and hands raised to engage with the opponent. The opponent is imagined to be walking on the opposite side of the circle, or perhaps in the center of a circle. During partner practice, each player extends the forward hand and maintains contact with the similarly extended hand of their partner; meanwhile, the other hand guards their own body. When combined with the system's various hand changes, the nimble Bagua stepping method enables an immediate about-face and reversal of direction on that same circular pathway.

In contrast to Bagua, in Tai Chi Chuan the opponent can be considered to be on the outside of the circle while at all times the tai chi player maintains the hub or center position around which the opponent revolves. In contrast to Hsing-I, in Tai Chi Chuan the response to an opponent is dictated by the line of attack and actions the opponent undertakes and is usually less angular than the Hsing-I applications.

Each of these "internal" styles uses a different strategy and line of attack to deal with an opponent. Consequently, each style has a different emphasis on training methods. Each also has certain postures and applications which are unique to that particular style. Moreover, within each of these internal disciplines, there are also sub-styles or schools which have developed distinctive variations as to how things are done. For example, in tai chi, the main styles are generally considered to be Chen, Yang, Wu/Hao, Wu, and Sun. Each presents unique variants that are characteristic of that style.

• *The Internal Art of I-Chuan*: The name I-Chuan (*Yi Quan*) means "Mind Boxing" and its training methods include uncommonly long periods of standing completely still while holding certain shapes or postures. It is not as old and not as well-known as the other three internal martial arts. It was developed in the 1920s by Master Wang Xiangzhai (1885-1963), as an outgrowth of his earlier studies in Hsing I Chuan (Xing Yi Quan). Master Wang was born in Hubei province near Beijing and was a student of Hsing I under Master Guo Yunshen.

One of the underlying principles of I-Chuan is that a practitioner should use the most straightforward and simple way to get things done. Nothing too complex or fancy is considered necessary or useful. Such a method of martial arts interaction immediately appealed to me as it seemed consistent with my studies of Lao Tse's philosophy.

I-Chuan training consists of two main components. The first part is *Zhan Zhuang* ("standing pole/standing like a post") in which static postures are held for prolonged periods to develop awareness and cultivation of the natural internal energies of the body. The second part, *Shi Li* ("testing force/challenge strength"), consists of movement exercises that are done with a partner to make use of and apply the internal energies developed during the standing work. A person well trained in I-Chuan will learn how to use the mind to connect to his or her physical power.

In line with its simple philosophy, I-Chuan's *Zhan Zhuang* training method was also quite simple. Simple but not easy. Quite the contrary. It was a definite challenge. In the classes I attended, the student was required to hold standing postures for lengthy periods without moving. Sometimes this immobility could last for as long as thirty minutes in one position before changing to the next posture. As you can imagine, this can be exceedingly demanding both physically and mentally. During these long static poses, the accompanying instruction was to use one's mind to aid relaxation and to develop the generation and circulation of internal power. The training is designed to improve one's sense of central equilibrium. It is also meant to develop one's awareness of where unwanted tensions are accumulating and held in the body. Once recognized, such tensions need to be released. During any given practice session, the recurrent cycle of tension buildup, recognition, and release seemed endless.

The I-Chuan *Shi Li* system for partner work is very different from tai chi Push Hands training. Its two-person competitive exercise is called "join hands". I practiced this with Master Do on many occasions. Master Do didn't show much external action in his movements but he could certainly generate tremendous power. Over and over again, I would find myself thrown out in various, surprising directions.

I must admit that I was confused at first by this *Shi Li* method of applying one's physical power because I found the people who had trained in this manner were very strong but also very hard. Their bodies did not seem soft, yielding, and relaxed in the manner that tai chi advocated.

I was searching for the solution as to how "four ounces can move a thousand pounds". I hoped to learn whether there was a way to use the mind (*Yi*) without needing to use brute physical force (*Li*). Master Do assured me that *Shi Li* was a very practical method of martial arts training. Having faith in his teachings, I diligently practiced in the manner he prescribed.

• *An Inspirational Story:* Master Do told me a story about a demonstration he had witnessed where his teacher Wang Xiangzhai defeated a younger Japanese soldier in Beijing in the 1930s, maybe 1935. Master Wang was about 50 years old or so at that time and weighed just 55-60 kilos (120-130 lbs.). The soldier, who was skilled in both judo and kendo, was between 28-35 years old and weighed about 70 kilos (154 lbs.). The soldier had given a demonstration of his judo and kendo routines and had bragged about the superiority of the Japanese martial arts compared to the Chinese arts. He then challenged the crowd and offered to take on anyone who wished to fight him.

Master Wang accepted the younger man's challenge. The Master was not a particularly muscular person and was certainly much smaller than the soldier. However, the Master's tremendous skill and power were to triumph that day. At first, and to no effect, the Japanese man tried to use judo on the Master. Instead, the Master was able to throw his attacker and made him fly across the ring. When this happened, the soldier became quite angry; and, because he had lost face, he insisted upon having another chance. For the second encounter, the soldier wanted to change to kendo. The Master again accepted. But, being without a kendo sword, he said he would instead defend himself by using his long-stemmed, pipe. With the customary loud shout (*ki-ai*), the soldier attacked with great force. The older man deflected the attack with his pipe and again sent the soldier flying away. The appreciative crowd applauded enthusiastically when the Master ended the challenger's second attack so convincingly. When the match was over, the soldier knelt in front of the Master and apologized to him for being impolite, and requested that he be allowed to study with the Master.

Although this particular story was undoubtedly true, some other tales which are found in martial arts literature seem truly "fantastic". The feats described are highly unlikely to have happened and are quite unbelievable. Regardless of their credibility, such accounts often serve to inspire a person to practice their chosen martial art with more determination. To realize one's potential in the pursuit of any art form requires a certain amount of resolve and willpower beyond that demanded by life's ordinary activities. The inspiration provided by such anecdotes can play an important part in attaining such achievements.

• *A Return Visit with My Teacher:* After I had won the tai chi Push Hands tournament in Taiwan, I went to pay my respects to Master Do and to bring him a picture. He told me that he had learned to use his mind and not his strength when engaged in Western-style boxing and that was how he had become a champion.

I most recently saw him in Taiwan in April 2009. Master Do was then about eighty-five years old and I had known him for nearly thirty years. We had become very close friends over those years. I was treated like a member of his family and was often invited to dinner after we had concluded our practice. Master Do had two daughters, one older than me and the other younger. Often when I visited, the three of us would work together in the kitchen making dumplings for that evening's meal.

Master Do was a very spiritual person and I am particularly indebted to him for introducing me to the concept of *"Yong Yi; Bu Yong Li"*. This single idea came to be the driving force behind my tai chi journey toward the development of the soft way, my "Search Center" way.

◆ ◆ ◆

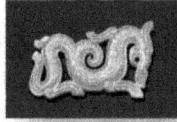

Chapter 5: The Malaysian Master

ALTHOUGH I HAD no way of knowing it at the time, the next tai chi master whom I met would be the man who would provide the key to resolving my questions about whether it was possible to reconcile the varied and occasionally contradictory tai chi teachings I'd encountered. The teacher was Grand Master Huang, Sheng Shyan (Huang, Xing Xian), (1910-1992).

He was born in Minhou County, Fujian province in mainland China. Starting in his early teens he had studied the Fujian White Crane style of martial arts and later learned other martial arts as well, including tai chi. In 1949, he moved to Taiwan. There he met and studied tai chi with Professor Cheng, Man-ch'ing. Subsequently, Master Huang was invited to teach in Singapore where he stayed for a brief period. He then decided to move to Eastern Malaysia, on the northern end of Borneo. Starting in 1959 and for the next thirty years, he lived and taught tai chi there and throughout south Asia. He eventually established twelve different school locations and today the number of students who practice his style of tai chi around the world is in the tens of thousands.

• *On a Visit to Taiwan:* In 1980, at the invitation of the National Tai Chi Chuan Association of the Republic of China (Taiwan), Master Huang attended the 4th Zhong Zheng International Tai Chi Chuan Competition in Taipei. During this gathering, a ceremony was held in which Master Huang was presented the gold medallion in Health and Sports by the then Minister of Education Mr. Zhu Han Sen. The accompanying certificate was presented by General Shi Jue, the Chairman of the sponsoring organization. This medal was given in recognition of Master Huang's untiring efforts over many years in the dissemination and popularization of tai chi.

At that time, I knew of Master Huang by reputation only. He was well regarded as a highly-skilled martial artist and teacher. I also knew he had studied with Professor Cheng, Man-ch'ing. I too had studied the 37 posture, Yang Style Short Form which had been developed and widely taught by Professor Cheng and then by his senior students. This lineage was something I shared in common with Master Huang.

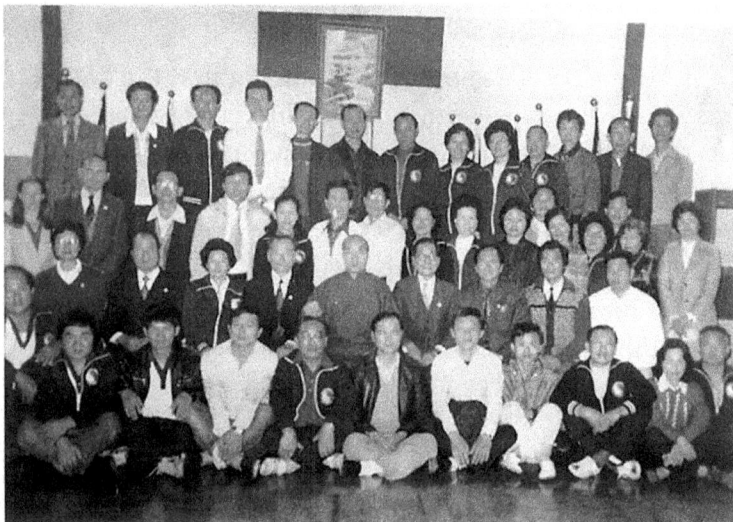

Master Huang, Sheng Shyan and Others
Annual Global Tai Chi Chuan Demonstration
November 23, 1980, Taipei
Henry Wang, third row, fourth from left.

Master Huang brought several of his students with him so that they could join the tournament as contestants. As it happened, I too was a contestant in that year's competition. Not long after I'd started my tai chi studies my teachers had encouraged me to enter various Push Hands events. I soon found that I was able to hold my own and even able to win my matches. By 1980 I had already won the Push Hands competition several times. During this 1980 tournament, I was also fortunate to win that title again and in doing so I had defeated one of Master Huang's students in a match.

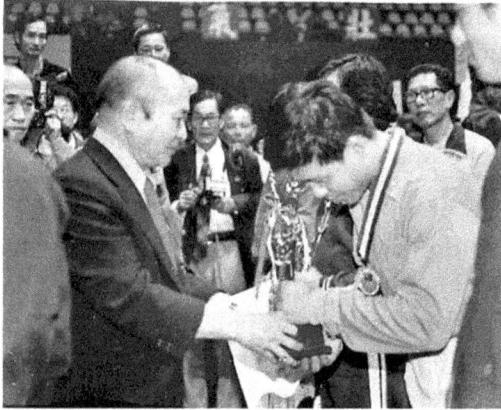

Trophy presentation to Henry Wang, 1980 Tournament.
Master Huang, Sheng Shyan observing, upper left edge.

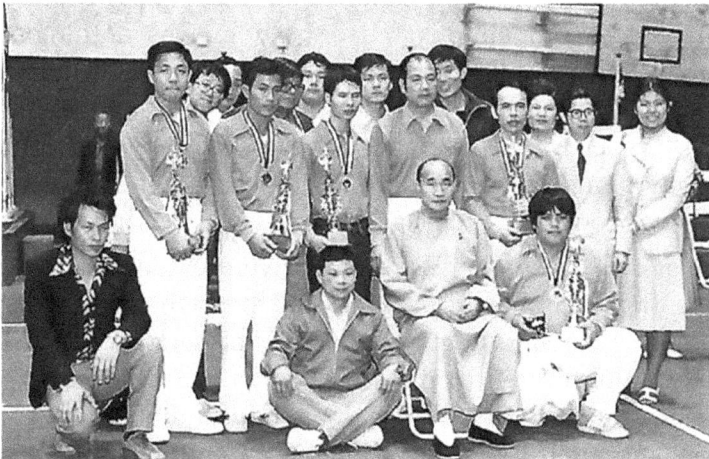

1980 Tournament Winners with Master Huang, Sheng Shyan
Henry Wang, Standing, First on Left Side

43

• *The Master's Push Hands Demonstration:* Through my years of participation in various Push Hands competitions I had become friends with Zheng, Xian Qi who was perhaps Master Huang's premier student living in Taiwan. Because of our relationship, I was invited to attend a tai chi demonstration which Master Huang gave during the tournament. This *"guanxi"* connection and karma would change my life again.

It was this astonishing exhibition by a seventy-year-old man that turned my tai chi world upside down. Master Huang simply took a normal, feet parallel, standing position with his hands loosely held near his chest, or in some other non-threatening, normal-looking shape. Each student would approach the Master in turn. Within an instant of reaching out to make contact with the Master, the student would be sent flying away, propelled across the stage by an all but invisible action. I could not see anything more than the slightest outside movement or a nearly token physical exertion by Master Huang yet none of the students could stand their ground or resist him. This happened again and again.

That such gentle gestures could have such dramatic results was beyond my experience. Certainly, what usually happened during the Push Hands competitions I had been in was nothing like that, including the one that had occasioned his visit. Push Hands matches were brutally quick and often depended as much on trickiness as on strength, speed, and leverage. All of which were attributes more routinely found in the realm of hard style martial arts even though tai chi was considered to be a soft style art.

None of those aggressive traits were evident in what Master Huang did. Yet the devastating and overwhelming effect of his minimal action was undeniable. Here I had seen for the first time an actual demonstration of the well-known phrase from the Tai Chi Classics, "four ounces can move one thousand pounds". I could not understand what I had just witnessed. Genuinely mystified, I was now even more curious and eager to learn how this was done.

Perhaps not surprisingly, many people who witnessed that demonstration did not think it was a true and honest presentation of martial arts skills. They felt that his students were just cooperating with their teacher. It did not occur to them that what they had seen was the effect of internal chi power.

By this point in my career, I had been at many tai chi competitions and demonstrations from north to south in Taiwan. I had never seen anyone move another person without actually using a physical push of some sort to do so, a muscle-based (*Li*) action. This was the first time I'd seen such a feat without the use of any hardstyle technique. To me, this was an occasion where I had witnessed a display of true internal arts proficiency. I was fascinated. I wanted my friend, who was one of the Master's students in Taiwan, to introduce me to his teacher as soon as possible.

Master Huang just worked with his own students during that Push Hands demonstration. Even though I was able to stand very close to the Master that day, I could not figure out how he was able to have this effect on them. There was so little movement on his part yet the students were immediately repulsed and thrown in any direction he chose. I was quite puzzled and wanted to experience for myself what it felt like to be tossed away with such forceless efficiency. However, I couldn't just step up and challenge him or insist that he must then and there do the same thing to me. To do so would have been considered extremely impolite. He was an esteemed guest and honored Master. I needed to show him nothing but friendship and respect and certainly not any confrontation or rudeness.

• *The Master's Tai Chi Form Demonstration:* On that occasion, Master Huang also displayed a brief segment of his performance of the tai chi solo form. To me, the most startling aspect of this form demonstration was how slowly he moved from posture to posture. The pace was so slow, relaxed, and steady that it seemed an entire minute would pass before one posture was completed. The Cheng Man-ch'ing style as I had learned it was practiced slowly, but it was not practiced in what I thought to be the extremely deliberate manner that Master Huang used. Indeed, none of my other teachers, all of whom were very accomplished tai chi players, moved at such a slow tempo.

At first, I could not see any benefit to what I considered the excessively leisurely pace which Master Huang set for himself. My own experience as a gymnast and my success in Push Hands competition had not prepared me for what I saw. After all, Push Hands required fast movement, not slow. At least I thought it did. The combined effect of his slow-tempo form and his "forceless" Push Hands demonstration left me walking away even more confused than before about what exactly constituted correct tai chi.

That day I also heard Master Huang talk about the need for tai chi players to develop their internal energy through the cultivation of increased relaxation, a state of being called "*Sung*". Relaxation he emphasized was very important to progress in tai chi. So, then and there, I decided to dedicate myself to becoming more relaxed in my tai chi practice.

Before meeting Master Huang, I had devoted a lot of training time toward the development of various Push Hands techniques and maneuvers which would allow me to yield and avoid the effects of a competitor's attacks. During his remarks that day, the Master urged everyone to learn to be soft and to accept any incoming push in a more refined and relaxed manner. He advised us not to resist the incoming force even though we would often lose the encounter. Under those circumstances, failure should not be looked upon in a negative light. Despite the failures, he assured us that each day our tai chi abilities would be improving by training in this manner.

Based on what I had seen him do, I decided that I should use his suggested method in all my subsequent partner practices. Even though I was a Push Hands champion, I now began to train in a way that allowed others to readily push me. I intentionally let others do this so that I could learn how to remain soft and non-reactive under these extreme conditions. My friends could not understand why I would want to do this and constantly teased me about it. However, I resolved to continue training in this manner because I no longer wanted to rely on thinking about which technique I should use to avoid or get away from an incoming force. I wanted to learn how to accept and neutralize these attacks in a soft way. I wanted to develop a different type of skill. One that I could connect with the natural way advocated by Taoist philosophy. I wanted my body and my mind to become soft like water. When a tossed stone hits the water, the water does not offer any resistance. It accepts the stone and absorbs it completely. The stone's force is easily engulfed. It drops harmlessly through the surface and is gone. It is overcome and immersed in the non-resistance it encounters, the emptiness of Yin. For the next three years my training efforts were devoted to that end and it took me that long to achieve the deeper level of relaxation which I desired.

• *Following the Master's Travels in Taiwan:* After that first astonishing and inexplicable encounter with Master Huang I resolved to devote myself to study with him whenever and wherever the opportunity arose. My principal reason for making this decision was that to improve my tai chi I felt that I needed a new challenge. I'd already been fortunate enough to compete and win at the highest levels of Push Hands competition and had begun to ask myself what was next. What new goal could I set for my tai chi life?

After 1980 Master Huang began to make annual visits to Taiwan from Malaysia but his schedule limited his stay to just a couple of weeks on each trip. During those stopovers, the Master would travel around the island giving tai chi workshops and demonstrations. I would take a leave of absence from my job and arrange my life so that I was able to attend and join in those events. For the next three years, many of my limited vacation days were set aside exclusively for those travels.

I was determined to become fully accepted as a devoted disciple of Master Huang. To demonstrate my sincerity, I would wait outside his hotel room starting at 5:30 a.m. I simply was there to be available to assist him in any way which might be necessary. This was my way of showing my genuine sense of purpose and my willingness to be humble in the hope of being accepted as a pupil of this accomplished teacher.

Over those years, a friendship developed between myself and the Master. When he came to Taiwan, he would telephone me and invite me to come to his hotel and join the assembled troupe. I was much younger than the others in the group who traveled with Master Huang during his visits.

Compounding my difficulties in learning Master Huang's methods was the fact that I spoke Mandarin and the Master did not. The majority of his group were from Southern China and they spoke with a heavy dialect that I could not always comprehend. Consequently, when he gave instructions to anyone, it took me nearly two years to even understand the words themselves let alone the full significance of their meaning. I needed patience and perseverance to learn enough of the dialect to be able to join the discussion. I believe my persistence in all these things also demonstrated to Master Huang that my attitude toward the study of tai chi was not merely casual but based on a sincere devotion to mastering its principles to the best of my ability.

During those three years, I never saw Master Huang do the whole, solo tai chi form from start to finish. I only saw him do a few postures at any one time. Similarly, I received only a few words of direct instruction from the Master. Like other pupils, I was expected to observe and copy and thus learn how to become relaxed. How to achieve that particular qualitative state of being in the body/mind known as "*Sung*". To be instructed in this manner was the traditional Chinese way of teaching, especially in the martial arts. Observation and imitation were to be undertaken until the lesson was either learned or it wasn't. It either sunk in or it didn't.

During those visits, Master Huang would show all of us various relaxation exercises. He taught us how to drop our arms while turning the torso and shifting the weight from one rooted foot to the other. The work often involved doing just one drill or another repeatedly, time after time, over and over. But this training was much more than the tyranny of monotonous, repetitive motion. It was the requisite, principles-based discipline that is required of any athlete, musician, or artist who seeks to develop his or her talents. One of the other important lessons was to not move the hand independently from the body. In tai chi form practice the body should lead the hand; not the other way around.

The second year of my time with him he spent two or three weeks touring Taiwan. He would visit friends and famous people. I again took vacation time from work and made myself available to him.

• *A Lesson in the Soft Way:* By the third year, Master Huang knew my name. There were always lots of tai chi people hanging around wherever he went. One morning he called me to his private hotel room. This was my first chance to touch him.

I had been working steadily toward this moment and, given my tournament championships, I approached it with confidence as to my abilities.

We stood facing each other, each of us raised an arm and joined the back of our wrists. When I first made actual physical contact with him, I sensed he was very soft. There was no evident power there. Suddenly, I had lost my balance and found myself seated on the bed. I got up and tried again. Immediately and without delay, I was back sitting on the bed before I realized what had taken place. I had no chance and no choice in the matter. This happened perhaps three or four times in a row. And, just as quickly, our session was over.

I was stunned. In most tai chi competitions, I had a chance to react to the movements of the other player. Master Huang was so soft that I had no chance at all. None. My prior successes and whatever abilities I'd accumulated were of no consequence once I touched him. In each brief interaction, my skills were useless and ineffective against him.

There was no one whom I had encountered, whether teacher or fellow competitor, who was using the extremely soft methods that Master Huang was able to use so decisively against me and everyone else. My brief personal encounter with him made me truly believe that just as it says in the Tai Chi Classics, "four ounces can indeed move a thousand pounds". It was now even more obvious to me that to put this saying into practice you needed to be deeply relaxed and soft, to be truly *Sung*. I made up my mind to see if I could discover for myself just how this was done. After he left, I devoted myself to developing even more relaxation and softness in my practice.

In the fourth year, I received a telephone call at my home from one of Master Huang's students. The Master wanted me to come to his hotel in Taipei. Again, I took time off work and went to see him. By this time the friendship between the Master and me was growing closer. As usual, I arrived at the hotel early in the morning and waited outside his room until he called for me.

That morning he again showed me his set of relaxation exercises. How to drop the arms and relax while turning the body from side to side. Fortunately, this particular exercise and some other examples of Master Huang doing various relaxation exercises can now be found on the internet. These lessons have been preserved and presented for the benefit of anyone interested in improving their practice.

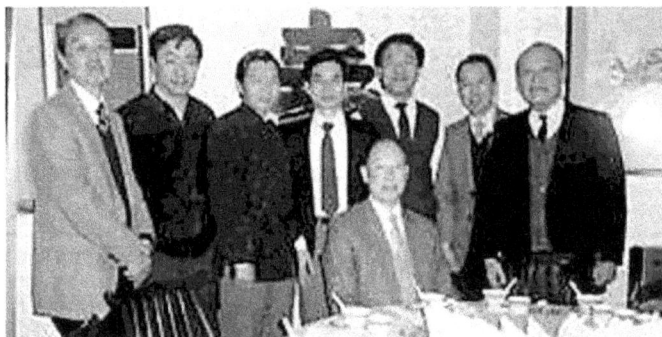

Dinner with Master Huang Sheng Shyan
(Henry Wang, third from right)

After that day's lesson, he invited me to join his group for breakfast. This was the first time I had been asked to share a meal with him and I considered myself very fortunate to receive such an invitation. For me, this was an honor in which to take pride. By this time, I understood his dialect better and was able to have a conversation with him during our meal.

• *Advice Regarding Push Hands:* During the several years I followed him, I did not receive any personal instruction directly from the Master regarding tai chi solo form practice. That did not bother or matter to me. I received, directly and indirectly, more than enough information to set me upon the correct path for the improvement of my tai chi, the development of tai chi's internal energy power, and the cultivation of *Sung*.

What I did learn from him I always found to be worthwhile, particularly his attitude towards Push Hands encounters. His advice was to let people push you and even knock you down. Do not resist those pushes; instead, try to neutralize them and thus make them ineffective. Your body and mind will become calm and relaxed from working this way. You will fail daily but you will also be improving daily.

So, I began doing partner practice work in this manner. Because I was trying to learn the soft way, I didn't care if my partner tried and succeeded to push me. I let them push me. My old tai chi friends thought that what I was doing was a joke and a mistake. They believed that Master Huang's students cooperated with him to put on a "good show" during a demonstration. Other masters whom I respected told me I was becoming too gentle and that Master Huang's methods would not work in a real fight. I believed my well-meaning friends were mistaken and that Master Huang's advice must be correct.

Master Huang told me to be soft and not use strength. I worked at doing so and my Push Hands became better. But partner work, even outside of tournaments, was still difficult because the Push Hands rules favored those who pushed. Pushing was how you scored points. Yielding did not earn points. (See Chapter 15, Push Hands & The Soft Way.)

• *Another Experience of Soft Power:* Master Huang always emphasized the health improvement benefits to be gained from tai chi practice. Additionally, he taught that if one became extremely soft in the practice then significant internal power would also be gained. One day, after Master Huang had conducted a tai chi demonstration, I had my first and only chance to practice Push Hands with him. I was truly surprised at how very soft the man was. As soon as I made contact with Master Huang, I felt as if my own body had suddenly become a rock sinking into the ocean. When I reached out and touched him, the Master immediately caught my balance and I instantly fell. Although I had seen him do this to others many times, it still was astonishing to experience. As I got up, I marveled at how remarkably easy it had been for him to suddenly drop me to the floor like that. This single episode taught me that achieving such a level of profound relaxation was critically important for building both the sensation of *"Sung"* and an acute sensitivity to one's opponent. After this encounter, I rededicated myself to working on my development of relaxation in hopes of attaining such a heightened degree of sensation and sensitivity.

• *Living a Simple Life:* Master Huang lived a very simple lifestyle. He got up early every day. He would be constantly on the go and would visit people all over the island. During these trips, I would often order his lunch for him. He did not drink alcohol. He did not even drink tea. He ate a simple diet, mostly fish, vegetables, and tofu.

One day he was giving a tai chi demonstration in a school. There were lots of tai chi groups waiting there to see him. It was a very hot day, even for Taiwan. The Master was wearing a long silver robe, a traditional type of tai chi apparel. I asked him whether it wasn't too hot to be wearing such clothing. He said that if your inside was calm and quiet you did not feel the heat.

On another occasion, I followed the Master to a demonstration in the southern Taiwan city of Tai Jung. It was an overnight trip. Master Huang had a large room with an extra bed. He invited me to share his accommodations and I was very pleased to accept. As further evidence of his preference for leading a simple life, the Master wore just a t-shirt and pajama bottoms to bed. He did not have fancy bedclothes.

• *A Few of Our Conversations:* We would talk at night about his experiences.

The Master told me that when he first moved to Malaysia he lived in a very small village. He would feed the monkeys, chickens, and other birds in the area. He told me that by studying the ways of nature he was able to improve his tai chi abilities.

Before meeting Professor Cheng Man-ch'ing, Master Huang had studied Shaolin White Crane style gong fu and gotten quite good at it. He had already won second prize in White Crane open fighting competitions for Fujian province. But Master Huang felt his gong fu was not good enough and needed improvement. He said that is why he began to study with the Professor.

He also told me about the time in 1970 that he won a famous wrestling match with Liao Guang Cheng, the 45-year-old Asian Champion Wrestler. Master Huang, at age 60, again demonstrated his superb tai chi abilities by defeating the younger wrestler, 26 throws to 0. The donations from the event went to a charity for orphans in Kuching, Malaysia. Film excerpts from this legendary match can now be found on the internet.

• *A Remarkable Exhibition:* Upon his return to Taiwan the next year, Master Huang called and invited me to his hotel. We had become friends and we trusted one another. By then several others in his group knew me too.

During this trip, Master Huang gave a truly remarkable demonstration. He first had himself blindfolded. His students would then come up to him and try to push him without being detected. Of course, no matter how quiet and secretive the approach, each one of them was sent flying away. One of the would-be "attackers" was not Master Huang's student but he too was sent flying. I, myself, did not participate in the demonstration but I witnessed it.

• *Respect for His Teacher:* In one conversation with him, I praised Master Huang's skill, "You are so polite that you do not use your push but yet you feel so soft." Master Huang said that he did not care if people criticized him for being too soft. He said you can't use force. If you do, you will lose your center and balance. When faced with a skillful opponent, you will certainly end up like a stone dropped into water.

I continued and told him that I had watched numerous films of Professor Cheng Man-ch'ing's tai chi and I thought that he had surpassed his teacher's tai chi accomplishments. He said that a student is never better than his teacher. As was typical of this man, he was being polite and showing respect for his teacher. Of course, Professor Cheng had exceptional skills in other pursuits as well and was known as the "Master of Five Excellences" (painting, poetry, calligraphy, traditional Chinese medicine, and tai chi). However, to me, Master Huang's deference to his teacher did not present a true picture of things. It is my opinion that his tai chi abilities had indeed exceeded those of his teacher. But, even after attaining this high level of tai chi skill, Master Huang remained humble and was not conceited about his accomplishments.

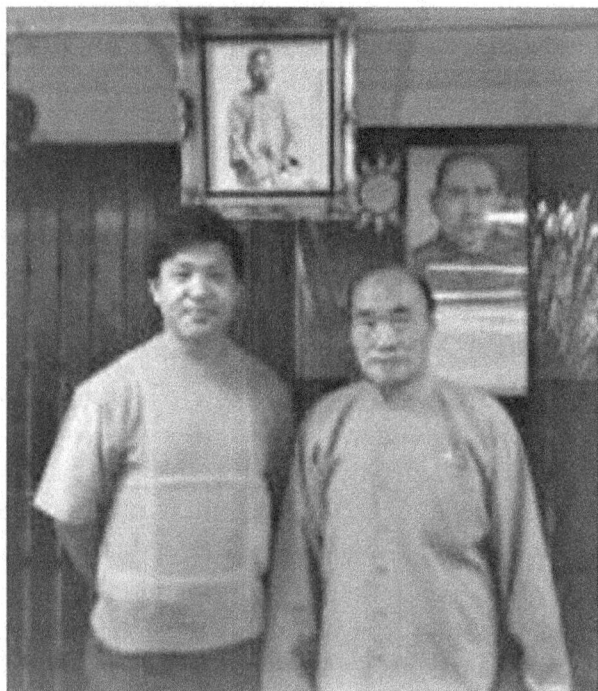

Master Huang, Sheng Shyan & Henry Wang

• *Documenting the Master's Tai Chi:* In 1986, the last year that I traveled with him in Taiwan, I urged Master Huang to record himself on videotape so that a record of his skills could be preserved for future generations. Very few people had video cameras then. They were just becoming popular and the prices were still too high for most people to afford. One of my friends, Mr. Su, happened to have one.

We all went to the Chiang Kai-shek Memorial Hall in Taipei to do a taping. This was the first time that I had seen Master Huang perform his entire tai chi form. I couldn't believe my eyes. It was so different from other tai chi forms and he performed it at a pace that I considered to be very slow compared to the many others I had seen over the years.

The following year, 1987, I emigrated to Canada and did not have the pleasure of touring Taiwan with the Master again before he died in 1992. Each time I met Master Huang over those years I realized more and more that becoming extremely soft in one's tai chi practice also results in one's tai chi becoming extremely powerful.

• *A Gift from Master Huang:* In 1989 Master Huang conducted a workshop in Belgium and invited me to attend. Unfortunately, I had other obligations that prevented me from being able to make the trip to Europe. After that Belgium workshop my friend, Ed, who was one of my students, came to Oakland, California to give a workshop there. Luckily, I was able to go down and meet Ed there.

When I arrived, Ed presented me with a surprise gift from Master Huang. Along with a personal note, the Master sent me a plaque and a photograph. I was deeply touched by this gesture of friendship and will always cherish his unexpected present. Both gifts have had a prominent place on the wall of my classroom ever since I received them.

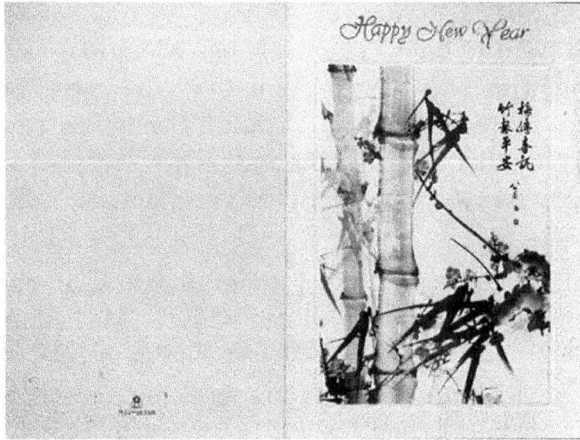

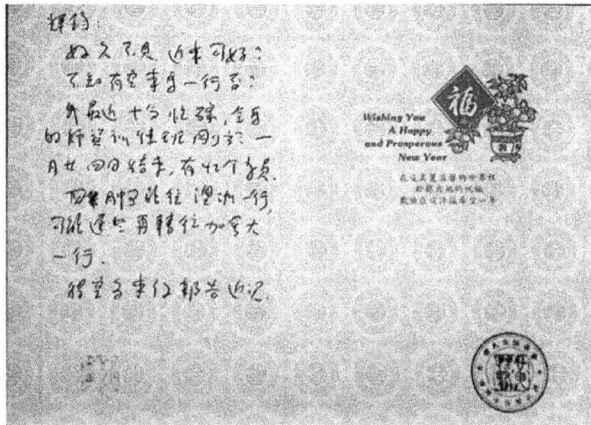

Among other things, the card mentions that Master Huang has not seen Hui Jiun (Henry Wang) for a long time and asks Master Wang to let him know how things are going. It also asks if Master Wang can come to Australia for a visit.

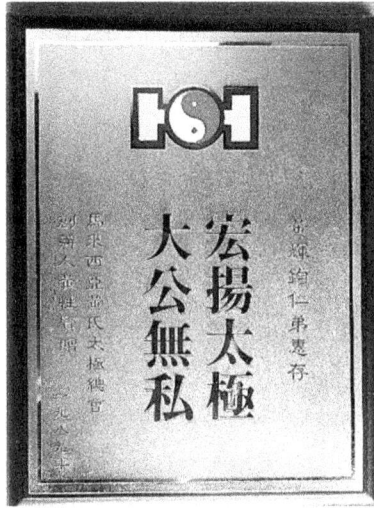

Gift Plaque from Master Huang, Sheng Shyan
to Henry Wang, 1989

At the top of the plaque is the symbol for Master Huang's tai chi school. The Chinese characters for Master Huang's last name and my last name are very similar.

On the right side, the plaque reads:

"Malaysian Grand Master Huang gift to Henry Wang".

The two central lines read:

"For promoting tai chi with great fairness and unselfish generosity."

The two lines on the left side read:

"Presented by Huang, Sheng Shyan, founder of Malaysian Huang Tai Chi, dated 1989".

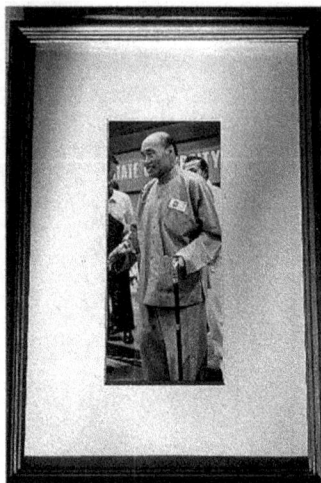

*Gift Photo from Master Huang, Sheng Shyan
to Henry Wang, 1989*

• *The Search for Common Principles:* To anyone who has practiced tai chi for any length of time it soon becomes obvious that there are several, indeed many, different styles. Chen, Yang, Wu/Hao, Wu, and Sun are the names of the five styles most widely known in the West but there are many other styles as well. Some are quite obscure and are only known and practiced by relatively few people these days.

Each of these different forms emphasizes different approaches to this art. For example, the Chen Style was often demonstrated at the competitions I attended. That style places considerable importance on developing power and using the form as an applied martial art for fighting. These days most tai chi masters do not accentuate the fighting applications of their particular style of practice. Instead, most other tai chi styles or schools that are involved in the competitive aspects of applied tai chi focus their efforts on training and preparing for Push Hands competitions. Yet a third group of practitioners focuses on the usefulness of tai chi as a practical method for improving vitality and increasing longevity. They see tai chi as being primarily a health-giving practice. These masters talk about how to become soft, pliable, and relaxed in one's practice.

Having seen these various styles and the different and occasionally conflicting lessons found in them, I became convinced that the study of tai chi should have some overriding principles. These principles would have to be shown to apply to all styles and practices. Then people would not be confused by the conflicting claims and methods put forth by the various styles.

I was certain that each of the tai chi masters I had met or studied with had ideas that were right in their way, but I was bothered by the fact that each master's training method was quite different. My experiences with them, and particularly with Master Huang, had inspired me to seek the most efficient way to train one's tai chi. I considered it extremely important for any such method to connect to and reflect tai chi's underlying Taoist philosophical principles. The method I envisioned should also contain and consistently reinforce three elements: tai chi philosophy, tai chi form practice, and tai chi's practical side as an art of self-defense. With those goals in mind, I began to reconsider and re-work everything I knew about the art of tai chi. After years of further study, trial and error, and continual refinement, I developed my Seven Principles for tai chi practice. (See Chapter 9, "The Seven Principles of Tai Chi".)

In establishing a sound tai chi practice, the student must develop good habits and adopt a consistent routine. Practice should become a daily occurrence but never a monotonous, mechanical, or mindless one. Another important aspect is that the student should maintain a humble attitude regardless of his or her level of achievement. There is always more to learn about the depths of tai chi. Even today I am still learning more about this art and striving to push my limits and understanding of what is possible.

◆ ◆ ◆

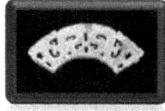

Chapter 6: Eastern Teacher, Western Students

ONE OF ITS unique aspects as a martial art is that tai chi has deep intellectual roots in Taoism. Taoist philosophy places considerable emphasis on impermanence, the constancy of change, and the harmony of the united opposites - Yin and Yang.

Before moving to western Canada, I studied Taoism and the teachings of Lao Tse for several years with Master Zheng, the retired philosophy professor. From him, I learned that as human beings one of our tasks in life is to accept and align ourselves with the variable and often turbulent nature of reality. Yet, resistance to change might be one of our deepest self-protective instincts. It is often difficult to accept and adopt change in any aspect of our lives. Nevertheless, we should continuously strive to maintain the right balance in life.

Although I brought those Taoist beliefs and other traditional Chinese cultural attitudes with me to Canada, I didn't realize at first how they might be tested. As it turned out, even late in the twentieth century, there were still occasions for cultural collision, confusion, and misunderstanding. As in centuries past, such episodes again occurred on both sides of the "East meets West" cultural divide. Thankfully, although feathers may have been ruffled on occasion, no real harm was ever done.

• *A New Preacher in Town?* Here's one example of just such a misunderstanding. In 1987, I left Taiwan with my wife and young family and immigrated to British Columbia, Canada. We first lived for a short time in a small coastal town near land's-end on the northern mainland. Then we moved across the Strait of Georgia to northern Vancouver Island and settled in the scenic Comox Valley where I've lived and taught tai chi ever since.

One day, not too long after our initial arrival in that small, mainland town, I made some flyers advertising my tai chi classes and posted them in various locations. Class schedules, prices, and my picture were included in the announcement. That same afternoon I passed by the posted sites again and was surprised to find that all my flyers had simply vanished and could not be found.

Later on, one of my students told me that he had heard that someone in town mistakenly thought tai chi was an Asian religion. The flyers had been torn down in protest of the new "missionary", dressed in his black suit, coming to town to preach. The "minister's suit" I'd been wearing in the photo was my tai chi silks, traditional martial arts clothing. I immediately laughed when the reason behind that incident was explained to me. Even now I am still amused by it.

These days tai chi has become better known to people worldwide and it would certainly not be mistaken for a religion. As for myself, I have never been a missionary or promoter in any religious sense. However, I suppose that my life's work is to some extent like that of a secular missionary if there is such a thing. The cause I campaign for is a simple one. I wish to bring the health benefits and enjoyment of this exceptional type of exercise to as many people as I can. Over some forty-five years of study and practice, time and again I have seen tai chi provide enormous benefits to my students, both physically and mentally. A consistent regimen of as little as ten to twenty minutes of correct practice, twice a day, can provide invaluable results. That is why I think it is so important that everyone learn more about the benefits that tai chi can offer.

Getting people to embrace the challenge of overcoming their inertia is the first and perhaps most difficult hurdle to reaching for that healthier life. Simply deciding to defy their ingrained resistance to make any change in their daily routines is a real problem for many. Old habits are hard to break even if a positive outcome is known to result. Indeed, the hardest part about learning tai chi may simply be making the sustained effort required to put a new habit in one's daily life.

• *An Apple for the Teacher?* The traditional Chinese calendar is based on a lunar system and not the Western world's solar-based method of calendar configuration. In the Chinese calendar, the day of a new moon is the first day of a new month. The Chinese calendar follows a recurring, twelve-year cycle and each year is associated with various animals, both mythical and real. People born in a particular lunar year are said to share the traits and characteristics of that year's animal. This idea is similar in many respects to the Western calendar's monthly signs of the zodiac and the various personality types associated with those signs.

In Chinese society, there are three, major annual festivals that have particular significance for the relationships within families and among friends. These events are related to the monthly lunar cycle.

The first and most important festival occurs in February. It is the Lunar New Year or Chinese New Year (a/k/a: the Spring Festival) celebration. This gala event traditionally runs for two full weeks. It

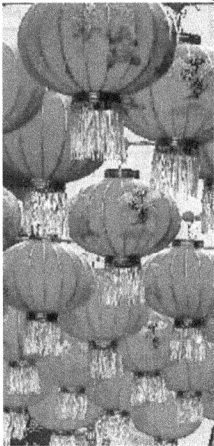 begins on the first day of the first month in the Chinese calendar and ends on the fifteenth day. This last day is called the Lantern Festival. Chinese New Year's Eve is known as *"Chúxī"*; it means "Year-pass Eve". Each year this festival is responsible for one of the greatest mass migrations of human beings on the planet. All who can do so head back to their hometown to celebrate with their multi-generational families. Unless you enjoy crowds, you might want to reconsider using public transport during this period.

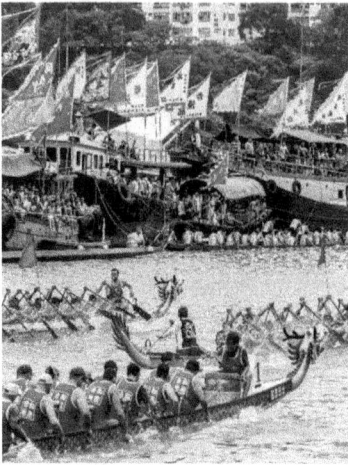

The second of these celebrations is the Dragon Boat Festival. It is held on the 5th day of the 5th lunar month of the Chinese calendar, usually in June. The Chinese call this day *"Duan-Wu"*. *"Duan"* means "beginning". *"Wu"* means "horse month". It commemorates the suicide of Chu Yuan (340–278 BC), who was a well-regarded poet and political leader in the state of Chu. It is celebrated on the anniversary of his death. In despair over inept officials and the invasion of his country by a neighboring state, Chu Yuan drowned himself in the Mi-Lo River. Each year, competitions are held among crews who race the well-known, long and narrow, dragon boats. Each boat is equipped with a magnificent and ferocious dragon head mounted on the prow. These races re-enact the frantic rush to save the drowning man. Tradition dictates that sticks of bamboo covered with rice be thrust into the water to feed the fish and thus prevent them from nibbling on his body.

The third celebration is the Chinese Moon Festival, also known as the Mid-Autumn Festival (*Zhongqiu Jie*). It occurs on the 15th moon

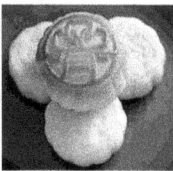

day of the 8th Chinese lunar month, around mid or late September. As this is yet another occasion for a family reunion, traveling at this time of year is again extremely crowded and chaotic. On the Moon Festival night, families and friends gather to eat a special moon cake pastry and admire the harvest moon.

One reason for the Moon Festival's contemporary popularity throughout China and Taiwan is that it has become the time of year when every company, large or small, gives each of their employees a gift of one-half of their monthly salary. Although some executives may get additional bonuses, everyone, regardless of rank, receives a gift of extra salary. It is given as a "thank you" for the hard work done throughout the year in making the company a success.

How does any of this relate to tai chi? For a student studying with a traditional tai chi teacher in China or Taiwan, it has long been the custom that he or she brings a gift to the teacher on each of these festive occasions. The cost of the gift is not of great importance. What is important is the attendant respect, devotion, and sincerity which is implied in the giving. This simple, thoughtful gesture serves as a demonstration to the teacher of the student's character and seriousness of purpose in his or her tai chi studies. It is a way of building a more cordial relationship between the teacher and the student and helps to strengthen their friendship.

Although I had attracted a fair number of students to my classes, during that first year in our new Canadian home there were no gifts for the teacher on any of those occasions. At first, I wondered, how could this be? Why didn't my students show the customary respect owed to their teacher? I then realized that this was simply an example of a clash between culturally based expectations. One that I hadn't previously anticipated. No disrespect had been shown or intended. There was nothing wrong. There was no one to blame. There was no real reason for me to be offended.

British Columbia is not China or Taiwan and northern Vancouver Island does not have the Confucian tradition as the framework for the dynamics of the teacher/student relationship. In my mind, I understood that our new home came complete with a new set of rules and expectations. Still, in my heart, I was a little surprised and disappointed that first year by this completely unintentional slight.

• *Reconsidering My Teaching Methods:* In Chinese society, there is a time-honored tradition of deference to one's teachers. This custom emerged from and was reinforced by the ancient Confucian ideal of respect for one's elders and the wisdom obtained from age and experience. This tradition was also reflected in the teaching methods adopted during the development of China's educational system.

That classical Chinese scholastic system produced eminent intellectuals and significant advancements in all fields of human endeavor, many of which predated similar accomplishments in the

West. However, what eventually developed in the classroom was a rather rigid, hierarchical structure. It was a top-down configuration that insisted upon obedience and submissiveness from each student. The relationship between teacher and student was clearly and inflexibly defined. Each had a distinct role to play. The student's part was the subservient one.

A dutiful pupil was expected to be quiet, respectful, and attentive. He or she was required to listen, observe, and copy whatever lesson the teacher was providing. The lesson was meant to be mastered and repeated more or less exactly as presented. Rote memory was highly valued, even in the absence of actual understanding. In a traditional Chinese classroom, questioning of the teacher's knowledge, or authority, or methods was not expected or allowed.

Asking a question was not considered to be an important aid to learning. The opposite was more the case. To question a teacher could be viewed as an impolite breach of etiquette. It was thought to be discourteous and a clear indication of a failure to show proper respect to one's superiors. Worse, it might even be considered an insult. To question a presentation was to perhaps imply that the teacher was inept, unknowledgeable, or unable to convey what needed to be learned.

This approach to teaching involves a point of view unrecognized in the contemporary classroom approach favored and prevalent in the West. The Chinese instructional practices were distinctly different from the Western tradition where a student's questions are seen as a sincere desire to learn and an opportunity to get clarification of points on which the student may be unsure. Since questions were not encouraged, dialogue with the instructor during class was nonexistent. Independent thinking on the part of the pupils was likewise not valued. A collaborative approach to learning was simply not the instructional model.

I understand that such restrictive educational methods have since changed in Taiwan, and to some extent in mainland China as well. However, it was this traditional Chinese method that I experienced during my school days.

What was true in an academic setting was also customary in the martial arts classes which I attended, only more so. No questions were allowed. The instructor would demonstrate a movement or posture and the pupils were expected to copy it faithfully, again and again, without question or complaint. The student's task was simply to observe, copy, and learn by doing. So, this was the "correct model" for instructional situations which I brought with me when I relocated to Canada and began teaching my tai chi classes.

Looking back on those early classes I sometimes wonder who was more shocked, the students or the teacher. Our expectations for how a classroom should be run were so different. There was not only a language barrier there was also a true cultural divide. I struggled with my English words and Chinese methods for some time as did my students.

Taking encouragement from my understanding of Taoist philosophy, I soon (perhaps some of my former students would say not soon enough) began to change my methods to fit the situation. Gradually, we all came to better understand one another. Nevertheless, there definitely were some miscommunications along the way, both in language and in methods.

• *Student, Disciple, or Customer?* In 1986, during my first trip to Canada, I started teaching a few tai chi classes in Powell River on mainland British Columbia and in the Comox Valley on Vancouver Island. Although the schedule was only temporary, the attendance was good and the classes were well received. When I departed for Taiwan, I left with the feeling that if I was able to return to Canada the students would return as well. In 1987, when our family made the permanent move to Canada and settled at first in Powell River, I resumed classes as soon as I could. However, it took me nearly two more years to come to a better understanding of what was for me a truly foreign and unfamiliar approach to the master/student relationship. I hadn't been able to figure out whether the people in my classes were my tai chi students or my tai chi customers.

In North America, the standard model for any instructional activity conducted outside the public or private school systems (e.g., lessons in dancing, skiing, cooking, piloting a plane, surfing, etc.) is that of a small business operation. The teacher is the entrepreneur/merchant, his or her knowledge is the commodity being sold, and the student is the customer. Moreover, the customer is always right! If the product isn't to a student's liking or questions aren't being adequately answered, or a student's thoughts and concerns aren't given due consideration, then the customer could simply shop elsewhere. I have certainly lost some customers (in every sense of the word) along the way.

One day I was in a restaurant and observed some young children who were upset with their parents' decision about something. To my astonishment, the children began to openly argue with their parents. They even called their parents terrible names and displayed evident contempt for them. It was then that I realized that in Canada the relationship between parent and child was on a more equal footing than in Chinese society. Chinese culture placed the parents above the children in all manner of things and such an occurrence would have been far less likely, particularly in public.

Once I had this insight, I was better able to understand the Western perspective on the relationship between student and teacher. While respectful, the relationship was also on a more equal footing. This realization made me feel more confident and self-assured in my evolving teaching style.

Those interested in learning more about how I came to live in Canada and made it my family's new home should read *"Flowing the Tai Chi Way: A Voyage of Discovery by a Tai Chi Master and His Student"* written by Peter Uhlmann, M.D., my most senior student. I first met Peter and his wife, Ronnie, in Taipei, Taiwan in 1983 when they began to study tai chi with me. In 1986 they invited me to visit them at their home in Powell River, British Columbia. They are the ones who enabled our entire family to permanently emigrate to Canada in September 1987. My wife Ivy, our two children, and I are so fortunate to have met our dear friends. We all highly value their many years of friendship, a friendship which has continued for close to forty years now.

• *Students Come and Go:* In the early years of my teaching in Canada, and even now to some extent, some students came to study tai chi out of simple curiosity. The merely curious did not take tai chi seriously. They were just investigating something novel. They soon left for the next fad.

I also had some students who faithfully studied tai chi with me for a couple of years and then abruptly left. They had come to class each week and diligently practiced the lessons at home each day. Suddenly, they would just stop coming to class without any further word or contact. I was at a loss to explain this change in their behavior. If I ran into one of these former students on the street or in the grocery store, I would learn that they were off pursuing another interest, belly dancing perhaps.

After several of these encounters with former students, it became quite evident that I should no longer harbor any illusions about the extent of the influence that I, as a tai chi teacher, would have on the lives of my students. In Chinese society, a teacher's power and ability to influence and shape a student's life beyond the classroom was well acknowledged, accepted, and appreciated. In my adopted country there was simply not the same cultural tradition or expectation.

On another occasion, a student who had studied with me for over ten years failed to return to the fall classes after the summer break. When I eventually was able to speak to him, I learned that he felt that tai chi had become too much of an obsession in his life. He felt that like a former drug addict or recovering alcoholic he simply had to give it up entirely. Naturally, I respected the student's decision even though I didn't fully understand it.

There were only a few students who saw and appreciated the many-layered depths offered by the study of tai chi. They were the ones who were interested in devoting themselves to the practice of tai chi as a genuine "lifestyle" choice and not just as a physical exercise or method of self-defense. They were the ones who returned to class regularly and who faithfully practiced each day.

What I now recognize is that each person comes to tai chi with certain ideas and philosophies of their own which they believe are right. The teacher cannot say "this is right; that is wrong". Each student must find his or her way. As their teacher, I try to share with them what I have learned in the hope that it will be of benefit.

• *Satisfied or Frustrated, Your Choice:* Perhaps one of the most common reasons that people drop out of tai chi is frustration. Tai chi, particularly in the context of Push Hands practice but also in solo form practice, can be one of the most exasperating activities ever devised. How so? Ego. For the most part, I do believe it is excessive ego involvement that trips up many a student.

Some students are drawn to tai chi because of its reputation as a highly regarded martial art. Tai chi literature is full of numerous glorious and inspirational stories. Among them are unlikely tales of masters jumping over the rooftop of an entire house. Events more likely to have occurred include the many, eye-witness accounts of triumphant masters who successfully bested all challengers. With the spread of video recordings on the internet, it is now possible to see historic footage of various legendary masters of the art. Many an old master can be seen instantaneously throwing about people who are bigger, stronger, and many years younger.

Some students come to tai chi because they want to attain those skills. They want to chase the power inherent in high-level tai chi. However, they often come with unrealistic expectations about the amount of "kung fu" (i.e., translated as "hard work") necessary to achieve the effortless power which the old masters can so easily demonstrate. They may not fully appreciate that what they are witnessing is the culmination of the talent, skill, hard work, and patient years upon years of practice which the masters have devoted to the cultivation of the art.

After only a couple of years of practice (barely a beginning really), these students get frustrated by their level of accomplishment or lack thereof. Their attitude changes: "I will never be like you, even if I do the hard work". This is the wrong attitude. The best reason to participate in any sport or exercise regimen is to promote and preserve one's physical and mental health. One should not compete just to score a victory or for the adrenaline rush involved. Those types of "thrill-seeking" athletes frequently take unwarranted risks, injure themselves unnecessarily, and even occasionally die at a young age. Instead, these students need to have more appreciation for the many health-related benefits of daily tai chi practice and learn to enjoy the cultivation of the tai chi way as an end in itself. Although a cliché, the "journey" is indeed at least as important as the destination.

• *What Does a Healthy Body Look Like?* The contemporary Western way of promoting physical health puts considerable emphasis on building strength, power, speed, stamina, and control. There is nothing inherently wrong with any of those attributes. They are just not the attributes that tai chi seeks to develop.

The tai chi idea is to relax and go the soft way. This attitude and approach are directly related to Taoist philosophy and its concepts of *"wu chi"* (emptiness as the source of everything) and *"wu wei"* (inaction; or perhaps more accurately, taking no unnecessary action; or taking only appropriate action).

I believe that in Western culture people have long been told, shown, and believe that a hard, fast, vigorous, and strenuous exercise routine is the proven and best way of attaining and maintaining a healthy body. They also want and expect to see immediate results from any exercise regimen they pursue. They don't understand how there could be any health-related benefits provided by the slow, gentle, and graceful movements of tai chi. They don't realize that great physical power can also be developed by practicing in this manner. They don't appreciate the benefits of working with internal energy. Indeed, they may have never heard of the concept of internal energy, let alone experienced it or believed in it.

The tai chi approach to building and maintaining a healthy body involves the cultivation of softness and relaxation during movement of the body coupled with a quiet yet focused and attentive mind. This idea has little credibility or acceptance in the Western approach to health-giving exercise. To some, it can even seem dangerous.

I had one student who ultimately abandoned his tai chi practice due to quasi-religious objections. He did not trust the soft way and instead felt that softness would allow evil an easy entry. I feel this student had an incorrect understanding of the underlying tai chi principles. In this instance, the difference between Eastern and Western ideas was not understood by the student. But I respected his decision and did not try to dissuade him.

• *West Meets East:* In the late 1960s, tai chi was still a very young and unknown discipline in the West. It was similar to acupuncture in that regard: an unknown discipline, of foreign origin, based on questionable assumptions, with incomprehensible methods, alien technology, and with an unproven track record in the West. Although practiced widely in the resident Chinese community, acupuncture was still illegal in British Columbia when I moved there in 1987. However, as Taoist philosophy maintains, things changed. Now acupuncture is not only legally and widely performed it has earned considerable respect and a rightful place in the practice of Western medicine throughout the world.

Similarly, tai chi is now widely recognized in the West even though it may not yet be fully understood or appreciated. In the United States, much of the initial exposure to and interest in tai chi can be traced back and credited to Bill Moyer's 1992 broadcast on public television, *"Healing and the Mind"*. That series explored the "mysteries" of traditional Chinese medicine and included a thought-provoking segment concerning tai chi and its benefits. Since that show originally aired, acupuncture and Traditional Chinese Medicine ("TCM") have become much better known and accepted by both patients and physicians. To an even greater extent, the recognition and popularity of tai chi as a health-promoting form of exercise is growing and participation levels have increased dramatically year after year.

• *Tea, Anyone?* In many cultures around the world, the preparation and consumption of tea is an important social lubricant among family, friends, and business associates. The Japanese tea ceremony is known worldwide as a refined ritual that embodies that culture's highest aesthetics. It involves the meticulous preparation and presentation of a finely powdered, high quality, green tea which is consumed and enjoyed in a beautiful and serene setting. English society also has its own rather ritualized behavior surrounding its customary afternoon tea. That tradition is in evidence today at the Empress Hotel, in Victoria, British Columbia where afternoon "high tea" is still served. The event is very popular and tickets for the daily occasion are often sold out. While the Chinese manner of enjoying tea is not usually as formal as that of the Japanese or English, it is nevertheless an extremely warm-hearted social occasion with protocols and preparation rituals of its own.

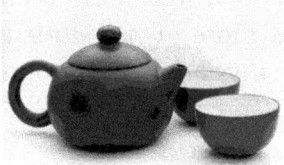

After our classes were finished for the day, I began to share with my students my love and knowledge of the various types of Chinese teas and the pleasurable social aspects of drinking and enjoying tea together while seated around the table. I introduced them to various varieties and types of Chinese teas: greens, blacks, oolongs, and white teas. We tasted freshly picked high mountain teas, aged pu-erhs, roasted teas, and fermented varieties. Spring teas and winter teas from Taiwan and mainland China were enjoyed as well.

This single plant, *Camellia sinensis* (the small leaf; grown in cool, high mountains) or *Camellia assamica* (the broad leaf; grown in moist, tropical climates) provides many social and health-giving benefits. The Chinese have known this for thousands of years and have been cultivating this plant and enjoying those benefits since first making this discovery. In our modern era, more and more Western scientific studies confirm the health-related benefits of drinking tea.

When I came to Canada most of my students were confirmed coffee drinkers. If they drank tea at all they usually added milk and sugar in the English fashion. The Chinese would never even think to add either to any of their teas. When I served it to them in the usual Chinese manner some of my students thought the tea was too bitter. They couldn't appreciate the unadulterated aroma, enjoy the mouth feel, or savor the pleasant, lingering aftertaste of a well-brewed cup of fine Chinese tea. Soon though, more and more of my students came to appreciate the subtle aromas and myriad flavors found among the many varieties of good Chinese tea. Following the Tao, they changed; changed from coffee to tea.

• *The Years to Come:* The growing popularity of chi kung and tai chi in the Western world and the increasing body of scientific knowledge concerning their many health-related benefits can be said to be following a path similar to tea's introduction to the West. Just as tea was first cultivated in China, so too the health regimens of chi kung and tai chi were first developed and widely practiced for hundreds of years only in China. As travel, commerce, and communications increased between China and the rest of the world, the practice of chi kung and tai chi began to spread to the West just as the tea market did.

Although gradual at first, these practices have now been widely introduced to the Western world thanks in large part to the growth of the internet. Although first treated with a certain amount of skepticism, the practice of these disciplines began to spread and the evident benefits soon appeared. Thereafter, the Western medical and scientific community began to look more closely at its effects. Their studies confirmed what Chinese medicine had long known. Soon the study and practice of chi kung and tai chi became more accepted and commonplace. Today you can find classes in nearly every city and participation continues to grow each year. Surely the health and longevity of people everywhere are being improved by their daily practice of these remarkable Chinese arts.

◆ ◆ ◆

SECTION TWO:

MY TAI CHI VIEWS & LESSONS

SECTION TWO

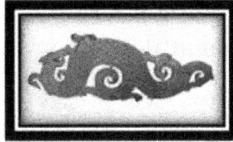

Chapter 7: Nurturing Fitness & Health

A S MENTIONED IN Chapter 1, when I got out of the army in 1973 I had begun to develop a serious interest in tai chi. In 1974, Ivy and I married and later our first child was born. After discontinuing my journalism studies, I took a job with a construction company to support my young family. The work paid our bills but my heart was not truly in it.

Since I was so dissatisfied and unhappy with construction work, I resolved to find a job that was more compatible with my lifelong interest in sports and physical fitness. I was certain that I'd be much

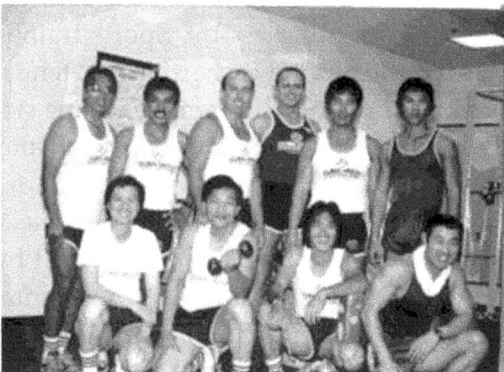

Fitness Center Group, Taipei, Taiwan
Henry Wang (front row, second from left)

happier in my work life if I were able to find a position that would allow me to pursue those interests and make full use of my athletic talents. After some searching, I was able to find a suitable position as a personal trainer and fitness coach with a fitness center in Taipei.

At that time, except at military bases, there were only a few such facilities in the entire country. The popularity of fitness centers for civilian workers was just beginning to develop. Soon I also became involved with fitness training for Taiwan's national sports teams and worked with professional athletes from various sports.

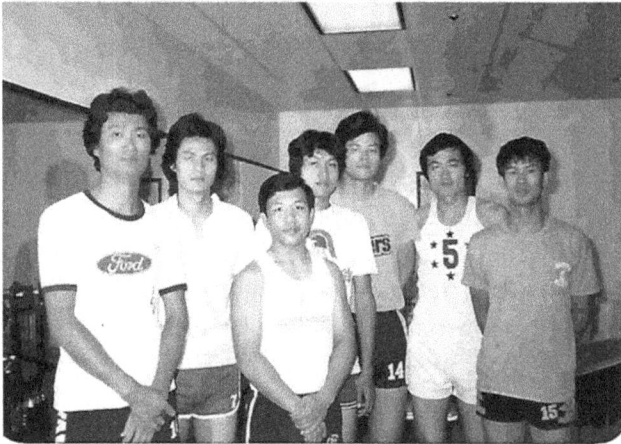

Taiwan's Olympic Basketball Team.
Henry Wang front row, center.

Tai chi as a regimen of physical exercise and training is completely different from other sports. Sports training, both in the Western sense and in the hardstyle martial arts, tends to place great emphasis on cardiovascular conditioning, building strong, muscular physiques, and training the development of speed and power. None of these qualities are actively sought in tai chi. Indeed, nearly the opposite is the case. Although tai chi can be performed with amazing rapidity and power those attributes are just useful byproducts and not the highest purpose of the training. It is the maintenance of one's health, physical, mental, and emotional, which is the higher purpose of tai chi training and practice.

Tai chi is a remarkable healing exercise for both the mind and body. If one is diligent in one's practice, emotions become calm, mental focus becomes more concentrated and one's physical body calms down and relaxes. The resultant composure and confidence, in turn, benefit the heart.

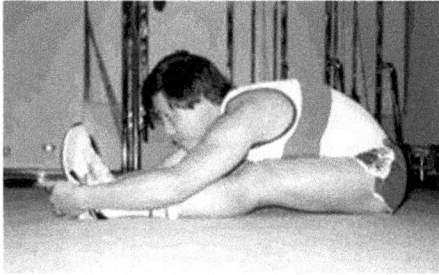

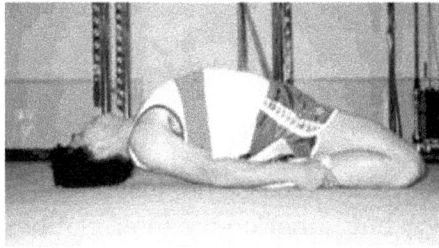

Henry Wang, Fitness Instructor

• *Tai Chi and Traditional Chinese Medicine:* I first acquired my deeper knowledge of the principles of Traditional Chinese Medicine ("TCM") after I had been pursuing my tai chi practice for several years. My daily hours of tai chi form work had been regularly supplemented with analyzing as many books as I could find about the various types of tai chi practices.

I soon learned that just as there is a natural association between tai chi and the principles of Taoist philosophy, there is also a similar connection between tai chi and the tenets of TCM. In the tai chi literature, there were numerous references to TCM and the effect of tai chi practice on building and preserving one's health. To better understand the interaction between tai chi, the cultivation and circulation of internal chi energy, and the principles of TCM, I decided that I should take up the study of acupuncture. Having successfully completed my studies, I obtained my license as an acupuncturist in 1975.

Nonetheless, it had never been my intention to start an acupuncture practice and I continued in my position at the fitness center, a job that I thoroughly enjoyed.

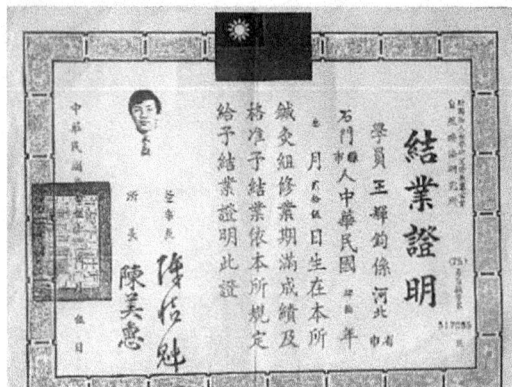

Acupuncture License, 1975

In TCM practice, the focus is not just on the individual, physical organs in the body but rather on the interrelationships and dynamic functioning of what is considered the various organ networks existing within the body. From my TCM studies and my tai chi practice, I have learned that tai chi simultaneously exercises both the inside and the outside of the body. In doing so, it aids in the more efficient functioning of the body's five organ systems that are described and explained in TCM.

For those who may not be familiar with the principles of TCM let me very briefly mention a few of its premises regarding the organization and functioning of the human body. In TCM there are five *"zang"* or solid organs (liver, lung, spleen, heart, and kidney) and a corresponding related group of five *"fu"* or hollow organs (gallbladder, large intestine, stomach, small intestine, and bladder). The complete system is known as *"zangfu"* and involves the interdependence of these organ networks. This *"zangfu"* system is also related to the Five Elements (wood, fire, earth, metal, and water) which in TCM theory constitute the basic elements or phases of the material world. The Five Elements themselves are considered to be in a state of constant movement and change. As depicted in this diagram, the outside arrows represent the cycle of generative change; each element leads to the next. The inside arrows represent the cycle of overcoming or controlling change.

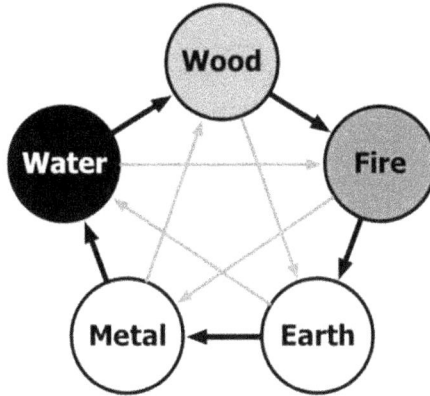

In Western medicine as well, the human body is considered to have various integrated and interdependent systems: respiratory, circulatory/lymphatic, digestive, endocrine, integumentary (skin), muscular, nervous, reproductive, skeletal, and urinary.

The overriding purpose of both sets of systems, East and West, is to maintain or restore homeostasis in the body. Homeostasis means the maintenance of potentially variable conditions within defined limits of functional acceptability. It involves many variables, including body temperature, hormone levels, rate of body metabolism, and fluid balance. The result is a healthy state in the internal physiological conditions of the body (and mind) in response to life's fluctuating conditions.

• *Tai Chi Practice and TCM:* It is well recognized that the regular practice of tai chi, preferably daily, can provide a variety of health benefits. Although tai chi originated as a martial art, its training routines are a type of mind-body exercise that can aid in the prevention and rehabilitation of a variety of health-related conditions. When done properly, its gentle, slow-motion, weight-bearing movements increase muscle strength and bone density. Yet, since the movements are low-impact they place minimal stress on muscles and joints. At the same time, the continuous motion involved while executing the various postures, coupled with the transitional movements from posture to posture, will improve a person's core strength, flexibility, and balance control.

Tai chi has been found to reduce joint pain associated with some types of arthritis, aids in fall prevention and reduces the risk of falls in older adults, can help lower blood pressure and can improve cognitive performance. In addition, tai chi practice reduces stress levels, aids in stress management, improves a person's mood, and has a positive effect on one's general health and overall sense of well-being.

My main reason for studying acupuncture was to improve my knowledge and understanding of tai chi and its effects on maintaining one's health. Daily tai chi practice does not produce immediately visible results even though it is extremely good for the health of the body's five organ systems.

For example, when doing tai chi attention is paid to keeping the hips horizontal. The knee joints are released (relaxed and slightly bent) and are not held in a "locked" position. One reason the knees are kept relaxed while doing tai chi is that in TCM the knee joints relate to the liver system. By keeping the knees relaxed the function of the liver system is improved.

In doing tai chi, an emphasis is placed on breathing from the lower dan tien level. This abdominal level of breathing is to remain quiet and unheard and never be noisy or labored. The breath should not be shallow but instead is deep. These various attributes of the proper breathing method for tai chi practice also promote the utilization of deep, abdominal breathing and are good for the body's lung system.

In tai chi, the development of a deep "root" in each foot is highly desirable and associated with the training of a person's balance and secure connection to the ground. By dropping the body's weight and allowing it to center into the "bubbling well" acupuncture point (*Young Chen*), just slightly behind the ball of the foot, one obtains a better balanced and more "rooted" stance. Such positional training stimulates that acupuncture point on the sole and thereby strengthens the body's kidney system.

In all styles of tai chi, the correct performance and execution of the linked sequence of individual postures always use a soft, circular pattern in extending and contracting the arms. Opening one's arms in this manner is good for the body's spleen system.

Regardless of the style of tai chi studied, the continuous performance of the tai chi form while maintaining a heightened awareness and concentration on the flowing nature of the movements from one to the next is beneficial to the heart system.

In tai chi practice we straighten the spine. In my own experience, this is good for the skeletal system and helps maintain healthy bones. TCM study bears this out as does my experience teaching my students.

Moreover, I have found that tai chi is not just physical exercise; it also is a regimen that is capable of healing the body. Among my students there have been many people who have sustained prior sports injuries. Often, after studying with me, their pain and soreness gradually diminished and they become stronger and experienced less discomfort or pain. Whereas doing other forms of exercise can lead to injury, their tai chi practice has been good for healing or alleviating the symptoms related to their old injuries.

A life of regular tai chi practice can also lead to prolonged health and increased longevity. Many tai chi masters have lived well into their 80's and 90's and some have even reached over 100 years of age. They also seem to avoid developing bad habits such as excessive drinking or smoking.

With so many types of exercise to choose from these days, why should someone choose to study tai chi? When I am asked such a question my response is that tai chi is the best method for self-healing that I know. From hundreds of years of human experience, we know that tai chi is a well-confirmed practice to improve one's health, rejuvenate one's body, and extend one's longevity. In my opinion, the regular, daily practice of tai chi can produce results that equal or exceed those obtained from other forms of exercise, or from taking expensive nutrition supplements and vitamins. Since tai chi is so good for health and healing, I would like to be able to share its many benefits with everyone in the world.

Whether viewed from a TCM and/or Western medicine perspective, the various health benefits provided by tai chi as both a preventive and rehabilitative practice is a vast topic and certainly beyond the scope of this book. I would encourage you to explore the many reliable sources readily available if you wish to learn more about this aspect of tai chi practice.

◆ ◆ ◆

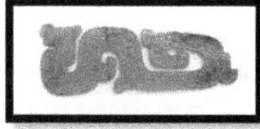

Chapter 8: Development of Internal Chi

MOST PEOPLE WHO are practicing tai chi today do not have any real understanding of its internal energy, its chi power. Despite numerous years of tai chi form practice, many have not recognized on a conscious level the distinct sensations occurring in their bodies as the internal energy circulates. Although chi is certainly present as long as they live and breathe, awareness of those subtle underlying sensations can be easily overlooked and missed entirely. Moreover, if the energy flow is blocked or has not been correctly developed the associated sensations will not have occurred. In turn, no truly "internal" work has been done during their tai chi practice. In the absence of such awareness and proper cultivation, little is gained beyond some physical exercise.

These people might have read or been told that the mind/intent (*Yi*) moves the chi and the chi moves the body. However, they don't truly comprehend the significance of that teaching. Even if they accept the assertion that the flow of the chi originates in the mind's intention, they do not understand how this happens. They have little or no idea of how to produce, cultivate or control this chi energy within themselves. Furthermore, they have even less of an idea of how to project this chi energy externally. They don't know how to use this chi in a way that will affect another person in either a "Search Center" or a Push Hands situation.

It is indeed regrettable that most tai chi players can do none of these things. As a consequence, their form is what I call "empty" and their Push Hands habitually relies on some combination of physical strength (*Li*), speed, and a plan for winning. By "empty", I mean that there is no accompanying presence of the internal chi which is originating and guiding their form's external movements. By "plan", I mean they have consciously chosen a particular technique to use or have a strategy in mind to win the encounter with their practice partners. Acting in this manner is inconsistent with tai chi's principles and philosophy.

• *The Three Dan Tiens:* To understand how to cultivate chi energy you should begin with the traditional Taoist idea that the human body has three dan tiens: an upper, a middle, and a lower. The dan tiens (tan tien, tan t'ien, dantian, or tanden) are considered to be the energy centers of the body, centers of life force or chi. The functioning of these three areas is interrelated and they must work in harmony for a person to generate better health, vitality, and mental clarity.

The upper dan tien is situated within the brain at a point on the forehead which is between and slightly above the eyebrows. It is sometimes associated with the pineal gland and is also called The Third Eye. The middle dan tien is commonly positioned in the mid-sternum region between the heart and solar plexus, in the area slightly above the diaphragm. It is regarded as the seat of emotional/empathic communication and regulates the body's Heart/Mind (*Xin*) connection, including the Spirit (*Shen*). But it is the lower dan tien that is considered particularly important and the primary area of interest in the art of tai chi. It is viewed as the body's main energy center and a focal point of tai chi's abdominal breathing methods.

• *The Lower Dan Tien:* The lower dan tien is located in the abdomen about three or four finger widths below the navel and approximately one-third of the way inside the body. In Japan, this region is known as the *"hara"* and the Japanese also consider it to be the seat of one's internal energy. Although this general area also contains the body's physical center of gravity and balance, the lower dan tien itself is not fixed in a specific, anatomical location. During a gross anatomy lab class, you cannot see it or touch it like you can an organ, bone, muscle, tendon, or ligament. Nor is it visible under a microscope.

In Taoist thought, the Five Elements symbol for this lower dan tien is that of water. Water has Yin (female/negative) energy. Another Taoist idea closely related to the lower dan tien is that of the heart/mind (*Xin-Yi*) which has Yang (male/positive) energy. The related Five Elements symbol is fire. In Taoist thinking, the task becomes how to unite these two, opposite yet complementary, internal forces (water and fire) to produce a third energy in the lower dan tien. The related symbol for the result of this successful unification is steam.

Interestingly, as long ago as the Han dynasty (206 BCE–220 CE) the Chinese character for rice was added underneath the older, previous character for chi (which meant air or breath) so that the combined symbols then indicated steam or vapor arising from cooking rice, the result of the union of water and fire.

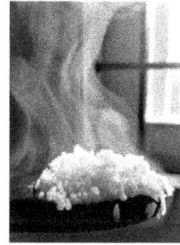

There is another straightforward analogy regarding the desired unification of the lower dan tien's internal chi energy. Consider a simple battery. Yin energy is the negative pole. Yang energy is the positive pole. Just as electrical current can flow only when both poles of a battery are properly connected, so too in tai chi. When the Yin and Yang energies in the body are properly harmonized the internal chi energy is then able to flow.

• *The Related Symbols:* The representation for how various combinations of this energetic harmonization take place is depicted via the use of the eight-sided Baqua symbols. The symbols are built using eight trigrams. Each trigram consists of all the possible combinations of any group of three lines, each line either broken or intact. When any two trigrams are combined, the result is sixty-four possible hexagram configurations. The Baqua symbols are usually depicted in one of two possible configurations; the one I prefer is shown.

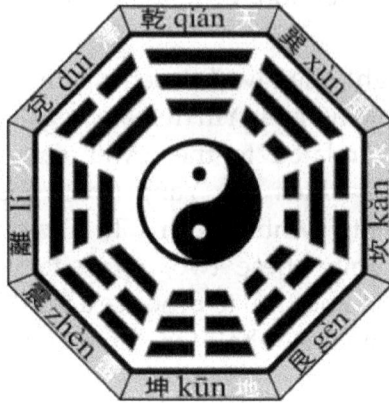

Fuxi "Earlier Heaven" Bagua Arrangement

Those familiar with the ancient Chinese divination system contained in the I-Ching or Book of Changes (*Yi Jing*) know that it contains sixty-four, oracular pronouncements each represented by a different six-line hexagram. Each hexagram contains a stack of horizontal lines divided into two trigrams. There are eight sets of these three-line trigrams. Each line of a trigram is either Yang (solid and unbroken) or Yin (broken and having a gap in the middle).

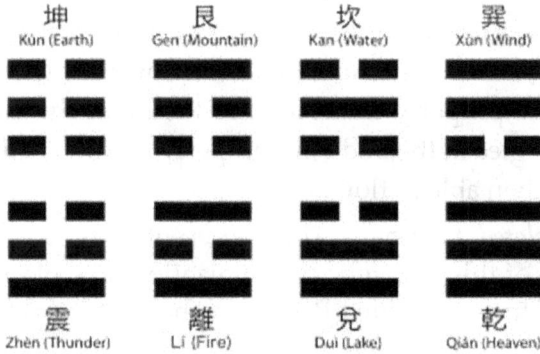

The Eight Trigrams

The union of the two forces of Yin and Yang is represented by the familiar tai chi symbol. The Yin/feminine side is dark. The

88

Yang/masculine side is light. Each has a small quantity of the other contained within it.

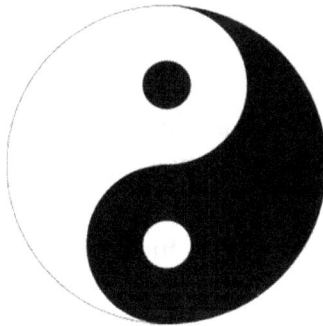

The Tai Chi Symbol

• *Daily Training of Your Mind/Intent:* That you can make use of your mind/intent (*Yi*) to develop your chi energy is thought by many people to be impossible. They are mistaken. It is possible.

To do this, you start by using your conscious mind/intent (*Yi*) to think about relaxing the physical body. Simultaneously, use water energy and related water imagery to help relax the muscles and let go of any previously unrecognized and now unwanted tension. Take a mental inventory of the entire body from head to toes. Where does it feel tight or tense and where does it feel loose and open? Release that newly perceived, excessive strain and tightness throughout the entire body. Then repeat the same body-state inventory and assess whether further relaxation adjustments are required. If so, correct again as needed. Continue these repeated assessments until you are reasonably satisfied that the restrictive tensions have been released.

Next, use the power of the mind/intent (*Yi*) to focus or concentrate on the lower dan tien. When combined with a comfortably relaxed body, repeatedly bringing your unwavering attention to this lower abdominal area will lead to the development and growth of your chi energy.

Although the practice method to achieve this goal can be stated simply, the discipline needed to accomplish the result may not be so easily acquired. The student needs to set aside at least twenty minutes of uninterrupted time each day. During this period, he or she will sit quietly, in a physically relaxed state, and focus his or her mental concentration exclusively on the lower dan tien.

The exact posture (standing, sitting, lying down) does not matter as the necessary concentration can be done from any position. However, it is probably best to sit on a chair or even on the floor, provided that you do so in a manner where the body is comfortably supported yet relaxed and without tension.

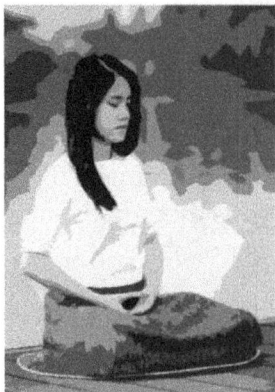

If standing or sitting, keep the spine erect, tuck in the chin slightly, keep the head as if suspended from above and relax the body. Do not collapse or slump. A calm, quiet, natural, abdominal breath should be used. Don't try to control your breathing. Just let the body breathe on its own. The key is to find a position in which you can remain immobile yet comfortable for the entire twenty minutes. If the body is properly and comfortably at rest it will be easier for the mind to focus.

Having attained a suitable posture, it is necessary to bring your entire attention, focus, and mind/intent (Yi) to the location of the lower dan tien and keep it there for the full twenty minutes. If you find that you are having difficulty, you can try a shorter period, perhaps no less than ten minutes though, and gradually increase it. The important thing is to start this training and then to persist each day.

To be successful, the mind's concentration must be complete in the sense of being steadfast and tenacious. The mind cannot be allowed to wander. Continual focus is essential. Just as in many other meditation traditions, the technique for disciplining the mind in this regard is simple to state. Each time the mind does wander it must be gently brought back to the task at hand without any accompanying self-criticism or blame. That's all. Maintain your awareness in the lower dan tien. If the awareness drifts (and it will) simply bring it back. Repeat this retrieval of focus as often as needed.

Although the instruction is simple, performing the task is often not as simple as one imagines. Determination and discipline will be necessary. Do not be discouraged. There is no set time frame for completing this phase of your development. Be prepared for sustaining your efforts and trust in the process. It might take as long as three to five years but do not shy away from undertaking the task. The rewards are certain to occur if you are willing to persevere in your practice. Based on my personal experience, I can tell you this is true.

When the mind and the lower dan tien join together, this is evidence of having achieved the first level of development of the internal chi power. However, most people are not patient enough in their practice. Rather than maintaining an upright spine and releasing and relaxing as much tension as possible in the abdominal area, they instead try to use force to achieve this connection. Invariably, they instead end up contracting their abdominal muscles. Regrettably, they won't ever get the correct internal feeling by acting that way. Instead, they just need to focus and concentrate while being quiet and relaxed.

From the Taoist tradition, we get the idea of how to accomplish this internal energy training. From the internal style of martial arts, we get the idea of developing the useful and practical, external expression of that internal chi energy.

Why does tai chi focus on the lower dan tien? The lower dan tien is the Yin part. The focused mind is the Yang part. For the chi energy to be expressed, it is necessary to produce the combined energy resulting from the union of both the Yin and Yang energy. That combination brings out a third quality which is greater and more powerful than the separate parts alone. A single Yin or a single Yang item working by itself will not operate at its maximum potential. The maximum potential is only realized when the female and male (Yin and Yang) are joined together. This potent third quality is an emergent property made possible by and resulting from their successful combination.

In chi kung practice, which is somewhat different from Taoist practices, meditation is also used to develop internal chi power. The breath remains calm as a means to let the body relax. Yin energy, like water, is used to develop chi power. The mind is used to drop the energy to the lower dan tien.

To many a tai chi student, there seems to be no tangible physical benefit in the short term to this mental practice of focusing one's attention on the lower dan tien area. However, with repeated practice over sufficient time, that lower abdominal area will begin to develop an internal sensation of heat or warmth. That subjective feeling of spreading warmth in the lower abdomen is indicative of the initiation of the internal chi power. It is a welcome signal that the internal chi energy has now become sufficiently accumulated and condensed for the chi engine to start up. The length of time required to achieve this varies from person to person; no general time frame can be reliably stated. The student should simply trust in the process and continue his or her practice.

• *The Microcosmic Orbit:* Once you have achieved the first level of attaining the sensation of chi in the lower dan tien, you then begin to use that accumulated chi to focus on other parts of the particular meridian channel which is called the "Microcosmic Orbit".

One of the goals of tai chi practice is to unify and enable the internal flow of chi energy throughout the two main energy channels located on the front and back of the body which comprise the "Microcosmic Orbit". The Yang channel (the "Governing Vessel/Du Mai") is located on the back. It originates in the lower dan tien and flows down to the base of the spine via a point on the perineum. It then ascends the mid-line of the back via the spine to the Crown Point at the top of the head ("Bai Hui" point). Then it travels down the front of the head where it ends at the upper part of the mouth and meets the Yin channel. Via a connection point located where the tongue touches the upper palate, the chi energy then descends the mid-line Yin channel (the "Conception Vessel/Ren Mai") on the front of the body and returns to the lower dan tien. The cycle then repeats.

92

There are several main points along this great circuit channel. Some points commonly mentioned are: the lower dan tien, hui yin (perineum), wei lu (tail bone), ming men (lower lumbar spine, about L2-L3, kidney area), yui gen (neck, Jade Pillow), bai hui (crown), mouth (yin jiao, closed mouth/tongue on the roof of the mouth) and tang zong (heart). The circuit then continues its path and returns to the lower dan tien where the energetic flow resumes its rotation.

As mentioned, to complete this circuit, it is necessary to have the tongue's upper surface lightly touching the upper palate at all times. In tai chi form practice you are likewise instructed to keep the mouth gently closed and the tongue in that position so the circulation of the energy can be maintained.

• *Filling the Kettle:* Most people are too eager to obtain the benefit of this circulation of energy and thus seek to circulate the energy before they have first developed sufficient chi for this purpose. They are like an empty tea kettle that is broken down and destroyed when put over the fire. Because it holds no water for the fire to boil, the fire instead consumes the kettle itself.

Likewise, if you do not have sufficient chi developed in the lower dan tien, when you focus your mind in an attempt to circulate the energy you will be like that waterless tea kettle; and, your efforts will not be successful. You shouldn't be hurried. You should not try too much too soon. You first want to fill the empty kettle of your lower dan tien with chi and this mind/intent (*Yi*) training is the proper method to do so.

As I mentioned, chi kung practice has a similar idea. Those practitioners also seek to generate chi power. But they do not include the concept of storing the energy which they have developed while doing their chi kung exercises. When they try to work with the energy, there is often too much fire while their "kettles" are empty.

In tai chi practice you first need bodily relaxation but the mind must also be focused to attain that feeling of warmth or heat in the lower dan tien. This is similar to Taoist teachings.

• *In My Classes:* When teaching my tai chi classes, I do not usually talk about the lower dan tien. Instead, I talk about whether or not the student's hands have become warm as a result of doing their tai chi form practice. Warmth in the hands is a sure sign of chi development in the lower dan tien. Even when practicing outside in cold weather, the hands should retain their warmth. Ideally, all the way to the fingertips.

Comox, my hometown, is located in the central portion of Vancouver Island, British Columbia. During the winter months, my students and I practice our tai chi form outside on most class days. No one wears gloves during these sessions regardless of the low temperatures and the occasional accumulation of snow on the ground. Even under such conditions, it is possible to generate sufficient internal energy/heat to keep the hands and fingers warm, provided there is no breeze to steal away the heat. Some students are more successful at this than others.

When I ask my students whether they have been able to keep their hands warm while doing the form many of them will answer no. As is true of other tai chi students, they are like incompletely filled "kettles"; they have yet to consistently develop sufficient water inside. However, if their hands are warm, then that is evidence that they have indeed developed chi in the lower dan tien. The more advanced students can feel their hands warm up but not necessarily every day. Some days the kettle will be full; other days it will be empty or only partially full. The student's task is to work toward filling the kettle each day, day after day.

The degree of warmth can also vary from day to day; that is normal. But if the hands, palms, and particularly the fingertips, get warmer during form practice that is a positive sign. You can't force this to happen. It is a natural result of improved chi circulation. When it happens, be aware of it but do not try to hold onto it.

On occasion, the warmth will come and go, perhaps more than once, while doing a single round of tai chi form practice. Other times, the warmth may only appear at the end of the form or at the end of several, repeated rounds of form practice. Sometimes your hands may get colder, even on a warm day. The student should always be aware of any such sensations and use them as a reliable indicator of the presence or absence of the chi's circulation.

There have been occasions when students whose hands have not warmed up attribute this lack of heat to not dressing warmly enough for the conditions, or they offer some other explanation or excuse. When students take that position, I generally just stop talking about chi development because such students are not listening. If you do the form correctly and with the right mental focus, the palms will become warm. This is a simple idea but the actual occurrence of this phenomenon requires a great depth of knowledge about tai chi principles and numerous rounds of form practice before you are likely to execute it properly and successfully.

This entire phenomenon relates to the saying I first learned from Master Do, the I-Chuan master, *"Yong Yi, Bu Yong Li"* (Use the Mind, Not Force.). My years of practice confirm the validity of this maxim. That such tremendous power can emerge from such softness is one of the remarkable mysteries of tai chi. (See Chapter 4, "The I-Chuan Master".)

◆ ◆ ◆

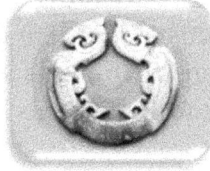

Chapter 9: The Seven Principles of Tai Chi
Universal Rules for All Styles

TAI CHI IS AN ever-evolving art. It always has been. It still is. Despite the deep-seated, Chinese deference to tradition and our cultural preference for honoring the past, tai chi has consistently generated new ideas and new approaches to exploring its various dimensions. As exemplified in the Yin-Yang symbol itself, there is an inherent tension in this dynamic between regard and respect for tradition and the need for innovation and change. In part, this is what makes the study of tai chi so interesting. There always seems to be more to learn, more to explore, more boundaries to challenge yourself with, and new answers to be pursued regarding the question: "What are the limits of this art?"

From its Chen family origins, several different styles of tai chi have emerged over the years. The Chen style has been followed by the Yang, Wu/Hao, Wu, and Sun styles for example. There is no denying the differences in both emphasis and execution, some subtle some not, which have appeared in these various styles from generation to generation. Moreover, even within any one particular style, different teachers have introduced their own interpretations and expressions of the teachings which their master presented. The resultant variety of approaches within a particular lineage can be confusing. Sometimes it is hard to recognize that these teachers were classmates who once had received a common transmission from their mutual master.

In the face of competing advice about the proper way to go about doing things what is the student to think? Beyond the universal admonition to relax, are there any common or shared elements that can transcend the obvious outward differences among the various styles of tai chi? Given this assortment of variations and their now and again contradictory instructions, is it possible to reconcile them? Achieving just such a reconciliation has been a passionate pursuit of mine for many years.

Now, with nearly five decades of practical experience to draw upon, it is my conclusion that a satisfactory resolution of this dilemma is achievable. The key is to first identify the correct, underlying principles common to all tai chi styles. Then, one need only sincerely pursue a practice regimen based on them. By devoting oneself to the embodiment of those universal principles, whether engaged in individual form practice or partner work, the student will ultimately attain the maximum health benefits and martial abilities that the art of tai chi provides. There are Seven Principles that I consider to be universally applicable to all styles of tai chi. Ranked in order of importance, those Seven Principles are: (1.) Relaxation, (2.) Center, (3.) Concentration, (4.) Circle, (5.) Proportion, (6.) Balance, and (7.) Coordination.

When doing tai chi form practice, it should be the goal of a tai chi player to embody all seven principles simultaneously. These essential qualities should certainly be exhibited in the final shape of each posture. But that is not enough. During every moment while transitioning from one posture to the next, they must be present continuously. Throughout a round of form, like the ingredients of a great recipe, all seven must be blended to produce a harmonious and satisfying result. Faithfulness to the unification of these principles in your practice will lead to the development and cultivation of greater chi energy and more internal power.

I believe that these core principles are indispensable to attaining the highest levels of the art. In the following pages, let me present some thoughts about each of them.

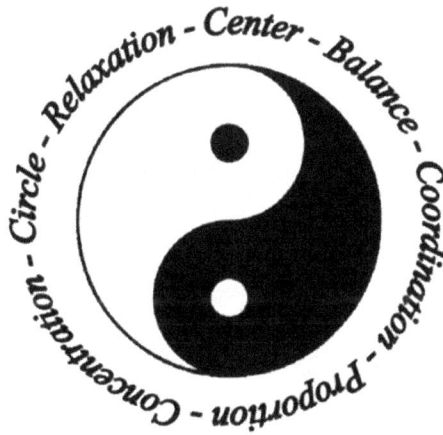

全身放鬆

Relaxation

1st Principle: Relaxation

I have placed Relaxation ("Whole Body Ease") first because, regardless of what particular style is studied, it is both the first instruction given to all students and the overriding characteristic and quality that all the other principles are designed to develop. From the outset, every tai chi student knows that achieving a state of relaxation is the often-declared goal for one's practice. A relaxed state is the condition most conducive to the cultivation of one's chi, the development of internal power, and the maintenance of good health. However, the essential components of that state or how to achieve it may not be well understood. It is neither very helpful nor nearly enough to merely have a teacher repeatedly scold you: "Relax! Relax, more! Just relax! Why can't you relax? Relax, relax, relax!"

Relaxation

What does it mean to be relaxed in your tai chi practice? Relaxation in tai chi practice involves achieving a highly refined state and harmonious balance of calm mental focus, correct situational awareness, and tension-free physical effort. The Chinese word for this state of physical relaxation, mental calmness, and attentive awareness is *"Sung"*. It is a qualitative state of both mind and body in which each is devoid of unnecessary tension, composed, tranquil, and resting in stillness. Yet, at the same time, the mind and body are fully present and responsive to their surroundings and environment. They are at ease, calm, alert, open, receptive, sensitive, "tuned in", and keenly aware of the slightest changes at the very moment they occur.

When properly trained, the presence or absence of this qualitative state manifests itself in certain physical sensations which can be felt, sensed, or experienced as they are occurring in your own body. Moreover, this qualitative state of relaxation can also be detected in the body of your partner during "Search Center" partner work. At the higher levels, this awareness extends to sensing and understanding your partner's mere intention to act/change before it is manifested in the actual action/movement of their body. Such highly developed *"ting jin"* (listening energy/skills) can ultimately be utilized for self-defense. (See Chapter 13, "Search Center".)

• *The Four Levels of Relaxation:* Everyone understands that there can be various types and degrees of relaxation in life. There are certain components of relaxation that are particular to tai chi. Tai chi practice works to develop a relaxed state that permeates one's entire being, both mind and body.

Relaxation in the context of tai chi practice can be divided into four levels. Level One, the most basic, is the relaxation of one's muscles. Anyone who has practiced tai chi for any length of time soon realizes that, although it may be the most basic level, it is not necessarily the easiest state to achieve. Level Two is an accompanying change in the body's tendons and joints; they begin to loosen and open more as the muscles learn to relax. Level Three involves an increased feeling of lightness, buoyancy, or floating in the upper body (above the waist/Yin) while the sensations in the lower body (below the waist/Yang) begin to feel heavier and heavier. The pelvis and legs feel solid, rooted, and well-attached to the ground. The lower body is felt to have attained a state of increased density or mass which is similar to that of a relaxed baby. When you pick up a relaxed or sleeping baby his or her body seems so much heavier and denser than its actual weight. Level Four involves a mental state in which the mind is calm and focused; it is fully present in the moment and neither tense nor anxious.

When you practice your tai chi form you are working at all four levels simultaneously of course but there are definite stages you go through in your tai chi development. Those steps tend to fall into place in the order I have set out. You begin by first releasing your muscular tension and then later you work on releasing your mental tension and anxiety. Optimum performance will emerge as each level becomes successively more and more refined.

Relaxation in tai chi practice is not passive. It does not come about as a result of doing nothing. It is instead a qualitative state of body and mind that is actively cultivated. What is particularly important about the principle of relaxation is that it can be practiced throughout the day in every type of activity that you undertake.

For example, how are you driving your car? Are you holding the steering wheel in a tightened, death grip? Is your breathing high or low in your body? Is your abdomen tense? Is your mind agitated? Are you angry or frustrated by the actions of those "idiots" around you? Are you wondering how they ever got a driver's license in the first place? When you pick up a hammer to drive a nail are you strangling the handle; or, are you so rigid and tense in the arm and shoulder that the effect of the blow is lessened by the surrounding muscular tension? When you swing an ax to chop firewood do you let gravity and the weight of the ax do most of the work for you? In any public setting, a cocktail party perhaps or a speaking engagement, are you confident or not? Are you worried about your clothing and appearance or whether your haircut conforms to the latest trends? All these daily events are just examples of signals that will tell you whether your body and mind are relaxed or not.

• *Relaxing the Mind in Form Practice:* I think it is generally agreed, at least in the developed world, that all of us are over-stimulated today by an intrusive flood of media of all types relentlessly clamoring for our attention. We are constantly being urged to multi-task our way through life. To be able to relax the mind in such an environment is a welcome relief. But how to do it? Relaxation of the body will be of direct benefit in producing a more relaxed state of mind as well. Thus, be unwavering in your resolve to train according to the Seven Principles each day.

As you work through the postures of the tai chi form, one aspect of mental relaxation comes from the combined focusing of intention (aim, goal, target, objective, plan) and attention (notice, concentration, thought, awareness, interest) to just the immediate task at hand. The mind does not always comply of course. Particularly during the beginning stages of your training, the mind will surely wander. It may even surprise you how frequently it does go off on some unrelated tangent. When it wanders, all you need do is recall it to the task at hand and resume your focus. Since you will need to do this repeatedly, this self-correction should also be done in a relaxed way. Reject any negative comments or feelings that may accompany the self-correction. Negativity can be counterproductive to achieving the calm and relaxed mental state that you want. Instead, correct yourself kindheartedly. Do so without blame, fault-finding, or negative, self-criticism. Perhaps the best attitude to adopt when you find that your mind has wandered elsewhere is one of amusement rather than frustration at your lapse of mental discipline. Treat yourself and your inevitable mistakes "softly".

In the form practice I advocate and teach, you first turn your Center, take an empty step, and then shift the body's weight. In doing so, pay attention to whether your body is relaxed. If you can release unwanted muscular tension, the upper body weight will feel light and the mind will become clear. If you can keep your mind in the dan tien, the back and stomach will feel heavy. The feeling of relaxation becomes equal throughout the body and the body feels securely anchored to the ground. Attaining a *Sung* state in both body and mind produces more chi; and, because the body has become more supple and coordinated, the body can move effortlessly, thus allowing the chi to move freely as well.

• *Relaxing the Mind in Partner Practice:* Partner practice is invaluable. It can be conducted in either a cooperative/ collaborative manner or an uncooperative/competitive manner. In either situation, it furnishes a reality check on the merit and usefulness of the work which a tai chi player has done in his or her form practice. It has often been said that if one's Push Hands practice is deficient both the cause and solution can be found in one's form practice. The same is true concerning the practice of "Search Center".

Partner practice offers a chance to test how relaxed you are in a more challenging situation. Even my most conscientious and hard-working form students express surprise when they first encounter partner practice. A gentle and cooperative "One-Hand Circling" exercise soon has them locked up in both mind and body. They become stiff and tense in their actions and anxious and apprehensive in their thoughts. Whatever degree of relaxation they had achieved in their form practice quickly deserts them and they are disappointed and frustrated by its disappearance. (See Appendix A for an explanation of "One-Hand Circling".)

This is a normal mental reaction to a loss of any type but it is not a useful one in your tai chi work. The solution to a state of mental relaxation in partner practice is no different than it is in form practice. You must keep your focus on the Seven Principles and your awareness in the lower dan tien. Ideally, you should be unconcerned about the outcome of any interaction. Simply do your best to maintain the principles. With your partner's help, you will find the solution to your awkwardness and your unnecessary and counter-productive use of strength. Indeed, you should always be grateful to your practice partner for offering you the chance to study and improve.

• *Relaxing the Body in Form Practice:* Physical relaxation, as found in tai chi instruction, is not what might be considered to be a state of relaxation to a Western student. The images surrounding a state of relaxation in Western culture might involve a hammock, a recliner, or perhaps a warm bath. It is generally portrayed as an inert and passive state. But physical relaxation in tai chi does not involve immobility. The relaxation we seek is not the same as lying on the beach or sleeping. The body in tai chi is not inert. It is involved in continuous and complex patterns of active movement. The movements become tai chi when they are done mindfully and with the least amount of strength and muscle tension necessary to perform the activity. The chest and belly must be released, the joints must be opened, the muscles, tendons, and ligaments, indeed the entire body, must become supple and coordinated. Be *Sung*. This is bodily relaxation in the tai chi sense. To do anything else is incorrect. Less is indeed more for once.

The body can accumulate and learn to carry a lot of tension. We can become so accustomed to this tension that it goes unnoticed. It becomes our normal way of going about our daily lives, full of unnecessary stress and strain. In tai chi, one must use the mind and concentrate on relaxing muscles and tendons. One must allow the body's chi to sink towards the ground. Relaxing and sinking the chi increases the development of one's root, that deeply felt connection of the body to the earth. Relaxation also allows one to listen better to incoming force and to use soft energy to overcome hard.

As I said above, but it bears repeating here, in your daily practice of the tai chi form you first turn your Center to move even one step; only then do you shift the weight. In doing so pay attention to whether your body is relaxed. If you can recognize and release any unnecessary muscular tension the body's weight will feel light and the mind will become clear.

Whenever practicing your tai chi form, in addition to properly composing a particular posture, there is a need to organize and connect the body during the transitions between one posture and the next. During the entire progression and slow, deliberate movement from one posture to another, you need to be constantly aware of your body's position and state of relaxation. You need to remain clear at all times about what the limbs and trunk are doing, as opposed to what you think they are doing. Is your body complying with the mind's instructions in the time and manner requested and required? Not just in the final position itself, but in each stage in the transitional positioning and in each moment along the way, you must pay attention. This is a Taoist idea concerning the maintenance of "attention/awareness" during physical relaxation.

Your tai chi practice should have the same state of wakefulness as that in seated meditation. Meditation is not sleeping. It is total awareness. Similarly, doing tai chi slowly and at an even speed enables better attentiveness to and control of relaxation. Just as you might watch a person who is meditating and not understand what is occurring beneath the surface, people watching you do tai chi probably do not understand what is happening to you internally while you move in this slow, careful and disciplined manner.

When you meditate, the mind becomes like a peaceful lake, shining and clear. If the air is still, there are no ripples; its surface remains calm and undisturbed. The water becomes so clear and transparent that you can see to the bottom yet the surface still reflects the clouds and sky. In tai chi movement, you want to cultivate a similar state of being. The movement principle in tai chi is to be calm, clear, and unhurried.

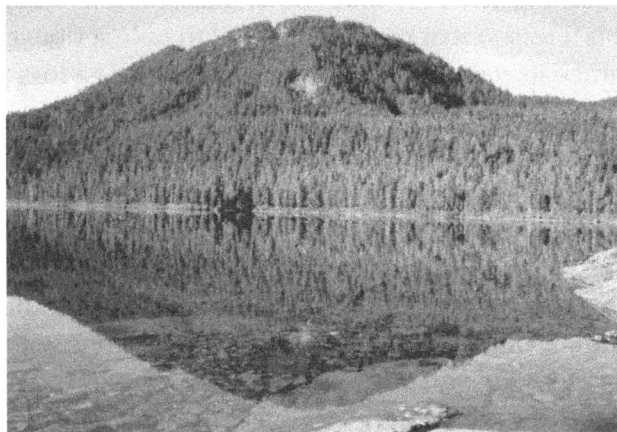

Using this or similar imagery can help you to become confident inside. It can be very noisy around you but you can become so focused that you don't hear it. You are aware of it but it doesn't disturb or break your concentration. Later on, this training will help you avoid becoming angry.

What is an essential feature of the tai chi art? The body in motion, the mind at rest.

• *Relaxing the Body in Partner Practice:* In solo form practice, you are developing and refining your ability to make the required shapes, continually increasing the amount of internal chi, and continuously improving the circulation of that chi. In partner practice, there are various stages in a student's ability to make use of the internal chi power which is developed during form practice. To make practical use of that internal energy when interacting with a partner it is necessary to give up the use of physical strength to achieve an effect.

This is the central paradox of tai chi, both in theory and practice. As you seek to reduce your reliance on the use of physical force against your partner, you will inevitably become more vulnerable to your partner's use of physical force against you. This can be a very frustrating experience and perhaps even cause some damage to one's sense of competence and self-confidence. It is easy to become discouraged. Don't let that happen. During partner practice, you must be willing to "invest in loss". This was Professor Cheng Man-ch'ing's training advice to his Push Hands students and it is still true today. It is a lesson that most people fail to take seriously. Or, if they do recognize its validity, they are nevertheless at a loss as to how to exhibit it in their partner practice.

To "invest in loss" does not mean that you should allow yourself to be easily unbalanced by your partner's actions. Rather, it means that you must learn to recognize your partner's incoming force and then make room within your own body to accept and welcome this force for as long as possible. You should seek to neutralize its effects by accepting it and allowing it through. This is done without offering physical resistance on your part. When you are out of room, simply yield. Accept the momentary loss of being tossed out as the price paid for learning how to neutralize effectively. Never offer resistance. Your skill level will gradually increase if you train in this manner.

To make relaxation in partner practice more readily achievable, it would benefit all students, whether beginning or more experienced, to divide partner work into two categories: cooperative/collaborative work and uncooperative/competitive work. Of course, there will be some overlap but that is okay. Why create this distinction? The principal reason is that the ability to use internal energy effectively requires the correct combination of "listening energy" (*ting jin*), right timing, and "intent". Since the sensations are novel and very subtle at first, in the early stages of training the student needs sufficient time to recognize what is required during a partner interaction. Training in a cooperative/collaborative manner reduces the tension and stress inherent in a confrontational setting and allows the participants to devote their full attention to the energetic aspects of their engagement.

We must remember that tai chi is a martial art and its postures contain excellent methods and techniques for overcoming an opponent in a situation that calls for applied martial arts. Particularly in the heat of competitive situations, internal energy can easily be completely overlooked. When it is missed, the student will instead revert to and rely upon some variation of a technique or an application that is inherent in the postures of the form. But, in the long run, it is those very techniques that must be sacrificed, de-emphasized, and even unlearned if one is going to gain access to the effective use of internal energy. I know this from my own experience.

• *Cooperative/Collaborative Partner Work:* There is much to be said on this topic; and, at this point, I will simply refer you to the chapter on "Search Center" which discusses this type of practice in greater detail. (See Chapter 13.)

• *Uncooperative/Competitive Partner Work:* This type of interaction is also essential to one's tai chi development because it teaches you how to relax the body and the mind when under attack via the aggressive use of physical force. The principal lesson to be learned is how to detect, yield, neutralize, re-direct, and/or absorb the incoming force. The initial and overriding goal in this situation is never to meet force with force or resistance. Meeting force with force will always result in the greater force overcoming the weaker. In tai chi, we do not take that path. We instead seek to soften and open the body in a manner that allows the incoming force either to pass by us and thus be avoided or to harmlessly pass through us and travel into the ground. In that latter situation, we are like a properly grounded lightning rod which allows the lightning to travel through and be absorbed harmlessly into the earth without causing injury. Practicing in this manner will eventually allow you not only to accept/neutralize the incoming force but also to return it effectively in a manner that uses your partner's force against him or her.

◆ ◆ ◆

立身中正

Center

2nd Principle: Center

立
身
中
正

Center

The Center (One Point of Origin) is the foundation that supports your tai chi form practice and form cultivation. It is the hub, axis, or pivotal point in the body from which all the internal spiraling movement originates. The Center itself has both a horizontal and vertical component and they must be joined together during form practice. To properly achieve this joinder, it is very important that the spine is kept straight and that the body not lean in any of the upright postures. Any discussion of the principle of Center should include some preliminary remarks about human anatomy and gravity's constant effect on our sense of balance.

• *Human Anatomy and the Center Point:* Anatomy textbooks customarily divide the human body into three cardinal planes and most of the body's movements are described as taking place in one or more of these planes. Simplified, they are the frontal, lateral, and horizontal. The frontal or coronal plane passes through the body and divides it in half from the front (anterior) to back (posterior). The lateral, median, or mid-sagittal plane passes lengthwise through the body and divides it into two halves, the left side and right side. The horizontal, axial, or transverse plane passes through the midsection of the body and divides it in half from the top (superior region) to bottom (inferior region), most commonly at the waist.

If you sketch a ball-shaped drawing with those three planes intersecting, the point where they all meet would also be similar to the area of your body's physical center of balance. This physical center of balance coincides with the lower dan tien area in Traditional Chinese Medicine and Taoist philosophy. It lies about three to four finger widths below your navel and approximately one-third of the way inside your abdomen from the front.

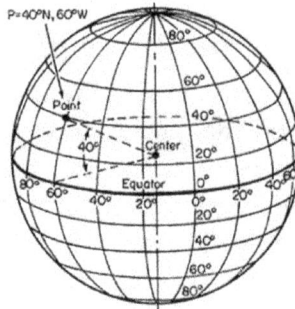

Center of Body Like Earth's Globe Shape

• *Gravity and the Centerline:* The principle of Center necessarily includes a discussion of gravity and its continuous effect on the human body's ability to remain upright. To state the obvious, everyone recognizes that the force of gravity is constantly acting upon us and keeps us attached to the earth.

While doing tai chi we should think about moving the body around a central, vertical axis which consists of an imaginary line that descends from the crown point (Bai hua point) on the top of the head, down through the middle dan tien, then down through the perineum (Huiyin point) and then still straight down into the ground. At the Beginning or Opening Posture of the form we stand with our feet parallel, weight evenly distributed on each foot, and the feet shoulder-width apart. In this position, the center of gravity drops from our crown point through the body to a single point on the ground directly between our feet.

If we maintain our shoulder-width distance but change the feet to an Archer's Stance [the front foot stepped directly ahead on a straight line and the rear foot turned out at the heel so the toes point at a forty-five (45°) degree angle] and have the weight distributed equally (50/50) on each foot, the central axis of the body still aligns itself with gravity via a pathway from the crown point through the perineum straight down into the ground between our feet.

If we next change our equally weighted stance by placing all of the body's weight (0/100) on the angled rear foot, the center of balance is "felt" to pass from the crown point on a line that descends vertically into the "bubbling well" point of the rear foot and then into the ground. Now, as we stand in that 100% rear foot position, an architect or engineer may draw the actual line of gravity slightly outside our bodies as it travels downward; nevertheless, in this particular rear foot tai chi stance, we are concerned with the felt sense of the body more than the true geometry of things.

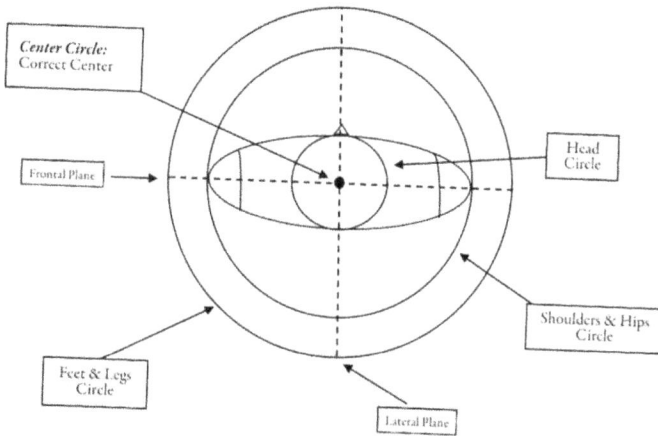

Overhead View, Correctly Aligned Center Posture

• *Center in Form Practice:* When I speak about the necessity of always maintaining your Center, I am speaking about having an ongoing awareness of a certain physical location in your body and the three planes which intersect there. This principle is not mine alone. The Tai Chi Classics advise the practitioner to "keep the mind in the lower dan tien".

When practicing your tai chi form you must maintain proper verticality in the upright postures so your balance will not be compromised. Likewise, in doing any of the non-vertical postures you must have a good understanding of where your Center (of balance) is located at all times. Without a well-developed sense of Center, you will be unable to maintain your balance properly.

• *Center as the Origin Point of Movement:* You must always begin any tai chi movement from your Center. It must start from there first. Then, just as the line smoothly unspools from a spinning reel when a fishing lure is cast, movement can begin to spin or rotate outward from this one internal point. Another simple analogy is that of dropping a stone into a very still pond. The ensuing ripples spread out evenly in all directions from the center point where the stone hit the water.

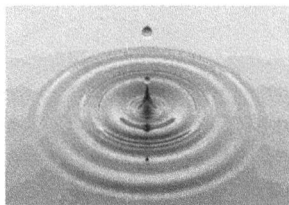

• *Center and Weight Distribution:* It is important to control your balance not only when the body is stationary but also throughout the transitions from one posture to another. This is how your tai chi root, your body's well-secured connection to the ground, will be developed. The development of your root is dependent upon and related to your practice of the tai chi form. However, in form practice, when working on your Center-based movements, there is more involved than just controlling your balance. You also need to control your weight distribution as you shift on your feet.

• *Center and Proportion:* In moving from the Center point you want to reposition your limbs in a manner that maintains an appropriate relationship between the major joints of the upper and lower body as you work to complete the transitions from posture to posture. The timing and position of the placement of the hands are related to the position of your feet. The same is true regarding your elbows and knees as well as your shoulders and hips. For more on this topic, see the later discussion regarding my fifth principle, "Proportion".

• *Turn First, Then Shift:* One of the untraditional instructions I give my students has to do with when to shift the weight while doing tai chi form practice. The traditional lesson is that the weight is first shifted onto the new foot before the torso is turned in a new direction. I was trained to move in that manner and spent many years doing so.

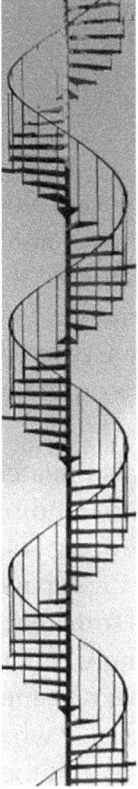

As the years went on and I gained more experience in working with the internal energy, I found this well-intentioned instruction to have been incorrect or at least not the best way to go about making any posture transition. Instead, I tell my students to turn their Centers slightly first and only after slightly rotating their Centers should they shift the weight.

The movements in tai chi are circular and spiraling. The chi coils around a fixed axis or center point like a simple helix shape. The internal chi originating from the lower dan tien emerges during the spiraling and rotational movements of the torso, joints, and limbs. To generate the most effective spiraling of the body's internal chi energy in an outward direction before the weight is shifted, the Center should be turned first. The Center leads all the movement. When you turn your torso first the Center spins and the spiral energy is both generated and then simultaneously released through the limbs.

It has been my experience that the trouble with the traditional "shifting first, then turn" instruction is that during the time it takes to shift the body into the new position one loses or disconnects the Center, which is the very source of the internal energy. If you follow the traditional "shift, then turn" method, the Center must be dismantled and then reassembled for each new posture. This causes a consequent interruption in the continuous flow of the internal chi energy.

On the other hand, if you instead "turn, then shift" your body's Center is preserved throughout the transition from one posture to

119

another. The internal spiral is maintained and the internal energy continues its uninterrupted flow. As illustrated in the "unreeling silk from a cocoon" imagery frequently used in the tai chi literature, there are no breaks.

"The Center Leads All Movement. Turn the Center First, Then Shift the Weight."

When form training is conducted in the manner I advocate, you will be able to discover and recognize where your Center is at all times. You will also be better able to detect and develop the continuous internal flow of the chi energy. Just as importantly, you will also be able to recognize when you are not properly Centered, and when the internal flow of the chi energy has been interrupted or is no longer occurring as it otherwise would.

• *Center in Partner Practice:* The Center principle is also related to my partner practice work which I call "Search Center". Finding and maintaining your Center is something that is done during solo form practice. Confirming that you have developed your Center and its related generation of the internal spiral of chi energy is something that is done during "Search Center" partner practice. For now, let me just say that to be able to find and connect to your partner's Center you must first start from your own. If you don't know precisely what being in your Center feels like and where your Center is at all times your attempts to connect with and control your partner's Center will be unsuccessful. More discussion about "Search Center" practice is found in Chapter 13 and Appendix "A".

• *Some Unnecessary Training Practice:* When I was a young man competing in tai chi tournaments, my colleagues and I thought physical strength was the number one requirement for success. Indeed, as part of our training, many of us included a daily weight lifting regimen. We even devoted considerable time to walking around the room while hugging large, fifty-five, gallon oil drums. To gain the most benefit from our workouts, we filled those drums with increasingly heavy amounts of sand or water. As the day's heat climbed and Taiwan's humidity became more oppressive those drums soon felt heavier and heavier. It was only later that I learned that it is the Center that controls whatever power you may have. The Center is the true foundation of your practice and the source of all power and balance. All that grueling, hot, and sweaty drum hauling we did was not needed.

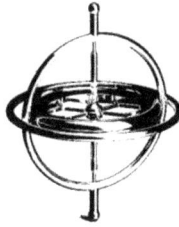

♦ ♦ ♦

専心一致

Concentration

3rd Principle: Concentration

專
心
一
致

Concentration

As a principle for proper practice Concentration has two aspects: attention and intention. It can be said that all voluntary movement begins in the mind. Whenever you initiate any action, you first have an idea that you want to do something that involves your body responding in a certain way. Pick up the glass. Kick the ball. Change the channel. Open the refrigerator.

This conscious decision that you now want to move the body to accomplish some task is different from an involuntary, spontaneous movement such as a reflex action (e.g., the patellar reflex which causes your leg to jerk when the doctor taps the tendon on your knee) or a sneeze or cough. The intent to act necessarily precedes the action itself. Interestingly, scientific research has recently shown that the body is already organizing itself to carry out an intended action before you become consciously aware that events are underway. The body itself commences the necessary preliminary signals and chemical responses incident to the initiation of the associated muscular responses that will be used to carry out that intention. Unless you intentionally intervene to stop the planned activity, it will take place as originally intended.

In tai chi, it is said that "the mind moves the chi and the chi moves the body". You have the intention to practice a posture, your chi flow activates the required systems, and the body operates to produce that posture. This sequence is obvious but it is so important that it should not go unmentioned. Why? Because with proper training, your mind can be used to direct the flow of chi in your body in such a manner that the circulation of the chi is improved and becomes more powerful. What's more, the mind can also be trained to use this chi to affect another person. The "Search Center" training methods I have developed will allow you to better understand how this works.

Whether doing your solo tai chi form or engaging in partner practice, having the appropriate intention at a particular moment or in a particular situation is not enough. The other aspect of the Concentration principle is attention or more accurately "paying attention". By this I mean the degree or extent to which you are aware of what is happening as it happens. Paying attention has numerous elements. It can concern your internal physical sensations, your emotional state, and your degree of proprioceptive awareness. Proprioception, also called kinesthesia, involves the accurateness of your internal sense of the external positioning of your body and its limbs in space at any given point in time.

During partner work, more of this attention is shifted from you and your external/internal state of being to your partner and his or her state of being. You focus more on what his or her body feels like to you when you first make contact with it (e.g., is it stiff and rigid or soft and yielding) and what his or her state of mind may be. Is your partner being aggressive and attacking or merely waiting patiently for you to make the first move? In partner work, attention becomes doubly difficult, if not more so. You are now monitoring not just your own body and its reactions but that of your partner and his or her reactions as well.

Once you can recognize and understand at the first touch the present energetic state of both you and your partner, an even deeper, more sophisticated state of awareness can be obtained. You can then develop the ability to connect with and incorporate the partner's body and energy with your own. As a result of this all-encompassing connection, you are now controlling one thing, the combined energies and Centers of both persons. Having done so, you will become more successful in neutralizing and controlling your partner's actions. It's a wonder that this can be done at all!

• *Concentration in Form Practice:* If you aren't actively engaging the mind throughout your tai chi form practice, your form will be "empty". The internal chi energy cannot be developed, harnessed, and used to provide the best health benefits. Without an engaged mind in your form practice, what you are doing is mere repetitive, physical exercise. Granted, it is good to exercise the body; but tai chi asks much, much more and offers much, much more. By "empty" I mean that the tai chi form's inherent, internal power will be lacking. It is necessary to join the mind and body together to produce that internal energy and to be able to effectively exhibit the external expression of its spiral power. When doing partner work, this absence of chi will also prevent you from developing the internal energy in a way that will enable you to use it to affect another person.

It all starts with training the mind. As the mind becomes more focused and relaxed the body will also become more coordinated, unified, and relaxed. Gradually, the movement patterns in the tai chi form become second nature, like riding a bicycle. But beyond that, gradually you will learn to use the mind to develop and move your chi. In tai chi, there are three levels to mental training: the Chi, the Yi, and the Shen. (See Chapter 13, "Search Center" for more discussion of this topic.)

The Chi level of your mental training, at least initially, involves developing an awareness of the existence and flow of the vital, "life force" energy that is constantly streaming through your body. There are a group of internal physical sensations commonly associated with this phenomenon. These sensations will vary from person to person and can be difficult to adequately describe in words. Typical descriptions can include a "tingling, buzzing, warmth, heat, etc." that occurs throughout the body and particularly in the hands and fingers.

The Yi or mind/intent level is the next component. At this next level of training, it is the intention formed in the thinking mind (*Yi*) which not only recognizes the flow of chi but also can influence and eventually control its flow to various parts of your own body on command. Additionally, the Yi can also use this chi flow to affect the body and chi of another person during partner practice.

The third level is the Shen or spirit level which is the deepest level of mental practice. It takes many years of discipline and training to attain that level of awareness and development. The result is that in any situation in your life you are better able to acknowledge and accept whatever is occurring without undue concern. This acceptance enables you to face events directly, cope with them effectively, and as a result, find the best solution to the situation that you face.

When you pursue any activity, whether tai chi or perhaps baseball, the training, practice, and study you undertake teaches you how to cope with novel situations as they occur. The discipline and concentration involved in systematic training allow you to develop the required skills and enable you to automatically depend and fall back on them as being reliable means to cope with any obstacles you face. The time spent training in the proper methods equips you for the given task and gives you confidence in your ability to meet the challenges presented.

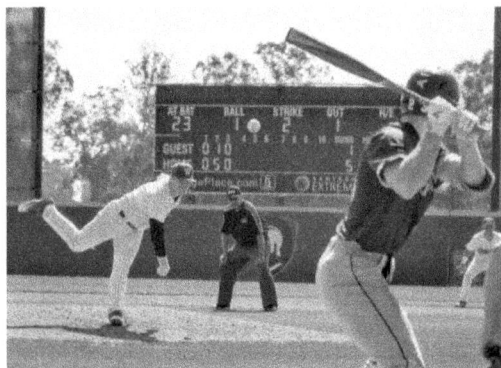

As when hitting a baseball, when practicing your tai chi, the mind must remain calm while simultaneously focusing on what you are planning for the body to do (intention) and on the kinesthetic/proprioceptive sense of what the body is doing at any given moment (attention). As in meditation, the mind must avoid wandering and instead continue to devote itself exclusively to choreographing the form postures according to the Seven Principles. The mind is capable of amazing power if correctly channeled. When properly cultivated, the mind directs the movements in the tai chi form as well as the searching of a partner's Center during "Search Center" work.

While doing the form (the external aspect of the practice) you are moving the physical body but your mental and emotional state (which are key components of the internal aspect of the practice) need to be still, quiet, and calm. Moving is Yang whereas being tranquil internally is Yin. These two aspects of the practice need to match. The Yin and Yang need to function and relate to each other as a cohesive, interconnected unit, just as they do in the familiar tai chi symbol.

Correct practice of the tai chi form will lead to a greater ability to concentrate your mind on the task at hand. When we start studying tai chi, the mind is caught up in learning how to make particular shapes and how to string them together in the required sequence; but even while struggling to do so, we will find that there is also lots of thinking about unrelated things. We distract ourselves from our assignment with random, irrelevant thoughts on completely unrelated topics. The mind just seems to go everywhere except for the immediate job we want the body to perform.

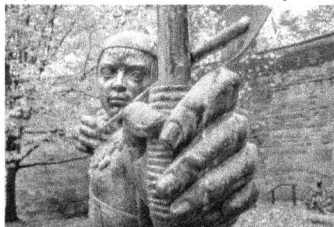

By practicing regularly and at a slow, even speed, we help the mind to focus and thereby improve our powers of concentration. At least three years of daily practice is needed before your mind becomes disciplined enough to truly concentrate during the entire sequence of postures contained in just one round of form. A productive session of early morning practice would ideally include three, consecutive rounds of form, each done with the requisite degree of concentration. You might set accomplishing three such rounds as one of your daily form practice goals. Resolve to be "present and attentive" throughout.

Once developed, you can bring this type of mental focus to any other daily activity. You become less distractible. This trait becomes even more desirable as our lives continue to be interrupted by electronic distractions and intrusions of every type. Multi-tasking is popularly seen as a virtue whereas current empirical research seems to indicate the exact opposite. Multi-taskers are not doing anything very well.

Tai chi form training will also make you more consistent and dependable in whatever else you do. The discipline obtained from maintaining a faithful practice, day by day and year by year, will carry over positively into how you handle your daily life.

• *Concentration in Partner Practice:* All your mental powers and physical abilities must be devoted to just one task when doing partner work, whether cooperative/collaborative or uncooperative/competitive. That task is listening to your partner. This skill is called *"ting jin"* or "listening energy". You need to focus on where that person's Center is and on whether he or she is about to unleash energy towards you. Just like you would sharply focus a camera lens or microscope to obtain the clearest image possible, in response to his or her intent you also need to be able to immediately focus your energy on just one point.

Having this level of listening awareness will enable you to respond promptly to whatever action your partner is intending to take. Indeed, when highly developed, you will be able "to read and respond" to his or her intention to act before their muscles have received the signal to act. There is a tai chi expression about "my opponent leaves first but I arrive before he does." This is what can result from such profound relaxation in the body coupled with the requisite calmness of mind. Since your body is relaxed, your muscles don't have to first unclench or stop doing one thing before undertaking a second thing. You can respond more readily and immediately, at the right time and right place to neutralize your partner's intention. Your attention, coupled with your proper alignment, will have made it possible for your body and chi to respond spontaneously as needed and with great effect. The relaxed body and mind allow the chi to flow freely.

◆ ◆ ◆

身形圓滿

Circle

4th Principle: Circle

身
形
圓
滿

Circle

There are several ideas involved in the concept of Circle ("Globe Shape"). The initial and most obvious one is that the chi itself is said to circle throughout the body along the meridian pathways many of which are themselves circular. The shape of the circle is present in all tai chi movements. The head circularly rotates on the spine. The turn of the waist and trunk involves a circular rotation. In the tai chi form, the postures are essentially circular. This is most evident when looking at the positions of the arms. The shapes they make are circular in many tai chi postures. When viewed from above three concentric circles can be drawn around the body. The first circle contains the head, the second contains the shoulders and hips (comprising the body's trunk), and the third contains the arms and legs.

Circles possess immense power. In the tai chi form, the Center turns in a spiral fashion. The chi energy comes up from the ground in a circular spiral around the limbs and trunk in its journey to the fingertips. After years of principle-based practice, the form's internal spiral becomes tighter and more compressed or condensed and the resultant power contained within it increases. This development of the relaxed yet powerful spiral energy assists the tai chi player to connect and circulate the incoming and outgoing chi. In "Search Center" practice the body can act like a large ball and incoming forces will seem to bounce off it.

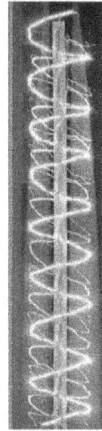

Constructing the desired "Globe Shape" in your form practice takes time. Once you have experienced the presence and flow of the internal energy trail during your performance of the form, faithful daily practice will gradually build up more and more energetic thread lines in the "Globe Shape" you are constructing around your Center. The process can be compared to the threads of silk spun by the silkworm in making its cocoon. More and more lines are spun until the structure is completely enclosed. Another circular analogy is the flow of electrons around the nucleus of an atom. The body becomes more unified in all directions. This is a gradual process. Just as you can taste the difference between a well-aged wine or Pu-erh tea and a similar but younger, less refined product, you get a comparable result from diligent practice over many years. Your tai chi will be a superior product.

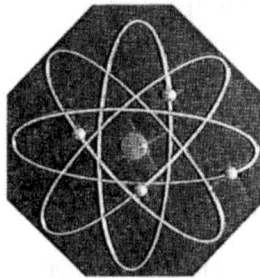

See the additional references to the "Globe Shape" in the remarks in this chapter regarding the fifth universal principle, "Proportion" and also the references to spiral energy in other chapters.

• *Circles - Opening the Joints of the Body:* For discussion purposes, it may be helpful to think of the body as having eighteen principal joints. There are four main joints in each arm: fingers, wrist, elbow, and shoulder. And four main joints in each leg: toes, ankle, knee, and hip. The final two joints are the neck (cervical spine) and the rest of the spine. Of course, the body has two hundred six bones and an even greater number of joints. There are as many as three hundred forty joints or more depending on what's being counted and who's counting. But for our discussion, the main joints of concern may be considered to be in the eighteen bone groups I have mentioned.

As a result of practicing the tai chi form, the body opens more and the body's joints get looser and more mobile. When the joints get freer and less restricted the circles of movement in the form become more apparent. As you practice your tai chi form and loosen each joint you will become better able to move that joint circularly. As you

134

progress and get even more limber you will discover a sensation that there are two concentric circles within the body, each having the same center point, one within the other.

You develop the imagery/visualization of the two circles. At first, there is a large outside circle and a small inside circle. At the higher level of tai chi attainment, the outside (visible circle) becomes small while the inside circle (the internal energy circle) becomes the large circle. This is easily seen in the actions of the old tai chi masters. Many internet videos show elderly masters such as Huang Sheng Shyan, T.T. Liang, or Ma Yue-liang making barely any physical movement of their bodies while sending much younger persons flying away. This is evidence of a very high degree of skill and accomplishment in cultivating the internal energy potential of the tai chi form. The previously smaller internal energy circle now has become dominant and is used by such masters to great effect during partner interactions.

• *Tai Chi Philosophy and the Circle Principle:* The Tai Chi Classics mention that the mind/intent (*Yi*) leads the chi and the chi's activation moves the body. The body's movement is, in turn, experienced and directed by the mind. This is a key cycle of tai chi practice. However, in tai chi, the concept of the recurring circle is not limited to just the circular shapes made by the limbs or the circulation of internal energy within the body. There is also a philosophical relationship between nature's cycle and the Tao.

The familiar sequence of the four seasons is perhaps the best example of a recurring, cyclical pattern. The rising and setting of the sun is another example of a circular pattern. Likewise, the stages of a person's life follow the circular pattern from birth, through childhood, adulthood, and then old age and death. If we practice our tai chi and use the soft way, we can slow this inevitable process of change and thus enjoy a healthy and prolonged life.

The tai chi principle of Circle includes tai chi philosophy. The Western idea of a healthy body usually emphasizes external conditioning and attributes such as muscle size, shape, and tone. In tai chi, we are interested in developing healthy bodies in a more sophisticated way and with deeper layers of meaning. The Western model equates the external look and function with health whereas the Eastern model looks more to the cultivation of the various internal organ systems of the body to assure they are functioning properly. In practicing tai chi, we cultivate a healthy body and we also cultivate a healthy mind by developing our powers of concentration and by observing the principles of Taoist philosophy.

In other martial arts, students seek to develop strength, speed, and technique. This strength will lead to more power and the ability to apply more force against opponents. The goal is to attain control over others and exert the student's will against their opponent's will. In tai chi, we strive to develop and use internal energy, to live in harmony with it, and with nature and with other people. We are not concerned with developing the power to control other people. This differs from other martial arts and certain sports which make use of force and power to dominate and control others. We should practice tai chi primarily for its health-giving and health-sustaining benefits.

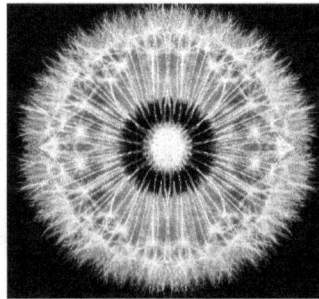

♦ ♦ ♦

左右對稱

Proportion

5th Principle: Proportion

Ratio, relation, relative amount, share, percentage, or fraction. All of these words are synonyms for "proportion". It has been defined as a part, share, or number considered in comparative relation to a whole. Or, as the correct or desirable relationship of size, quantity, or degree between two or more things or parts of something. When talking about a beautifully proportioned design it is said to be balanced.

Proportion

> *"To give something a pleasing shape, appropriate dimensions, or a harmonious arrangement of parts."*

This last phrase is perhaps the clearest statement of what this fifth principle, Proportion (Yin and Yang Together), entails. This is precisely what we seek to do when composing our bodies in any tai chi posture or while transitioning between them. If we can keep the proper ratios and relationships between the distinct parts of the body as we move through the form, we can generate a harmonious whole and not the awkward, clumsy, and graceless demonstration of disconnected parts so often seen. It is that harmonious whole that enables the optimum flow of chi and the maximum expression of internal power.

• *Constructing the "Globe Shape"*: One's tai chi posture should resemble a "Globe Shape" or sphere with the lower dan tien as its center point. The right hand is related to the left foot. The right elbow is related to the left knee. The right shoulder is related to the left hip. The same directive applies to the other side of the body. During the form, when weight is switched from one leg to the other, the opposite arm responds equally, proportionately, and in a synchronized manner. The arm opposite the weighted leg in effect acts much like a counterweight does in providing balance and stability while enabling more efficient movement. As more and more of the body's weight is gradually placed in the new foot, the opposite arm lifts and changes position at a matching rate while the mind/intent (*Yi*) directs the chi flow into the loosely extended fingertips.

One way to think about this idea of building the proportionate relationship between the opposite arm and leg is to imagine a hydraulic system filled with fluid. Increasing the pressurization of the liquid enables the generation, control, and transmission of power throughout the system. In tai chi, as the amount of compression is gradually increased (e.g., the body's weight is transferred from one leg's root and descending into the other leg's root), the power and energy are transmitted throughout the body and the chi spirals outward in the opposite arm.

Another useful analogy is the empty fireman's hose which remains flat and collapsed until the hydrant valve is opened. You can visualize the powerful stream rapidly coursing through the hose, inflating the entire length, until it bursts out the nozzle. Similarly, the pressure going into the weighted foot initiates the chi to flow like water through the body's open joints until it too comes out the arm and fingertips on the opposite side of the body. The pressurized limbs would be the Yang leg and arm. As they fill, their opposites empty at the same rate and become the Yin leg and arm. This is the embodiment of the idea of "cross-substantial" energy which was taught by Professor Cheng Man-ch'ing and others.

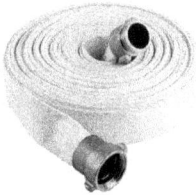

From my study of acupuncture, I know that the concept of providing a proportionate treatment is frequently used in caring for a patient. For example, treatment for a particular headache might involve work on the patient's foot as part of the healing therapy. In some instances of knee pain, the elbow joint may be the location included in the healing process. If there is pain on the left side of the trunk, the right side is where the needles may be inserted. Tai chi practice is also a type of healing exercise because its movements train and encourage a proportionate energetic response throughout the body which promotes the development and flow of one's internal chi.

•*Proportion in Tai Chi Postures*: In practicing the tai chi form it is important to strive for attaining the correct relationship in space between the various parts of the body, particularly the relationship between the fingers/toes, hands/feet. Take the posture "Brush Knee, Right Side" for example. In that posture, the right foot is forward. In making the shape it is important to develop the relationship between the action of the left hand and fingers as they come into the final position and align themselves with the right foot and toes. This is not an exact measurement done with rulers and tape measures. However, it does involve the correct shaping of the limbs in a well-timed manner so the increasing "pressure" sensation links the palm of the left hand and the sole of the right foot equally. Thinking about the Lao Gong acupuncture point in the middle of the left palm and the Yong Guan or "bubbling well" point on the sole of the right foot may help achieve the correct internal sensations.

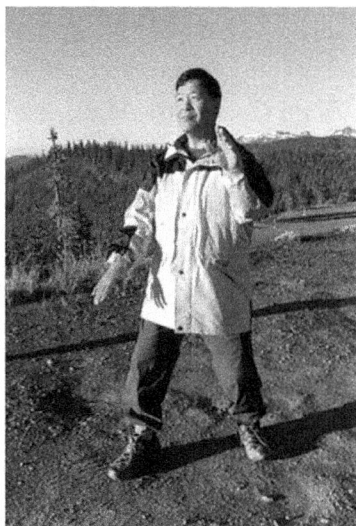

Brush Knee, Right Side
Master Wang, Summer Camp 2016

If you were to look down on the "Brush Knee" posture from above you would want to see the limbs contained within their respective circles. The hands should never reach out beyond the toes of the front foot. The hands should be positioned in proportion to the front foot. They should not be too close to the body and thus within the confines of the wrong circle. Similarly, the proper relationship between the elbows and knees should be maintained. Likewise, the relationship between the shoulders and the hips. One way to test proper positioning is to have a partner gently but steadily push against an arm and see if the chi flow is connected to the opposite foot.

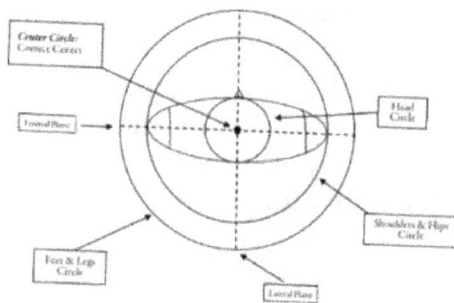

Overhead View, Correctly Aligned Center Posture

In your tai chi form, you want to move in a spiral that rotates outward from the Center. All your movements should start from the inside circle not on the outside circle. Turn the center and the trunk first, then the arms. "The trunk leads the arms.", I tell my students.

• *A Stop-Action Movie:* When performing any posture, it may help to think of your transitional movements as a series of frames in a motion picture. If you were to look at each frame individually (in "stop action" mode so to speak) you should see a consistent, proportionate relationship between the position of the arms compared to the amount of weight that is being transferred to the opposite foot. The increasing pressure you feel on the "bubbling well" point during a weight shift to a new rooted foot should signal a corresponding increase in the position, arc or curve, height, etc. of the opposite arm as it moves and articulates at the shoulder, then elbow, then wrist, then fingers. When this "movie" is played at normal speed the presence or absence of that proportionate relationship is easily overlooked. However, if watched in slow motion, the relationship or lack thereof will become more obvious. If you are interested and brave enough to do so, today's technology provides many ways to film yourself doing the form. Most cell phones can take a few minutes of video footage, enough to do one or more postures. Try filming yourself and then play it back in slow motion. I think you will be amazed at what you see. Your performance will certainly improve once you are aware of what needs to be corrected.

• *Center and Proportion:* In discussing Proportion, you must also consider the interrelated principle of Center. It is around the Center that you construct the proportionate relationship of the limbs. It might be useful to re-read the discussion of the Center and to consider these two principles as being intertwined.

In moving your body from the Center point, the hands and feet move together, the elbows and knees move together, and the shoulders and hips move together. We have all heard this many times. It is a standard instruction common to all of the various styles of tai chi. It is a correct lesson. However, we often lose sight of it during our form practice and are particularly inclined to forget about it when engaged in Push Hands or "Search Center". We are often so invested in defending our position that we allow ourselves to become distracted from embodying the very principles which will ultimately allow us to best protect ourselves, and to do so in a proper tai chi manner. I urge my students to be mindful of the Seven Principles during every tai chi activity and throughout the regular parts of their day as well.

◆ ◆ ◆

重心穩固

Balance

6th Principle: Balance

重

心

穩

固

Balance

Our sense of Balance (Poise in Motion) may indeed be our sixth sense. It has been defined as a state in which a body or object remains reasonably steady in a particular position while resting on a base that is narrow or small relative to its other dimensions. For people, this most commonly involves remaining upright and steady on the feet. Other synonyms are equilibrium, poise, stability, steadiness. Perhaps the most common symbol or representation of the concept of balance is that of a counterbalanced weighing scale like the familiar scales of justice.

The balance scale imagery can be useful when doing your tai chi form. As you turn your Center and shift the weight it may help to visualize such a scale. As the pressure increases in the weighted foot's "bubbling well" (Yong Quan point), can you notice whether there is an equal and corresponding increase in the energy in the palm (Lao Gong point) and fingertips of the opposite hand? While doing your form are you cultivating a state in which the various body parts match and form a satisfying and harmonious whole? Is the position of the limbs such that nothing is out of proportion or unduly emphasized at the expense of the rest of the figure? Is there a consistent equilibrium between the mind and body throughout the execution of a round of form? All of these are examples of the Balance principle and they are ideas closely linked to my Proportion principle as well.

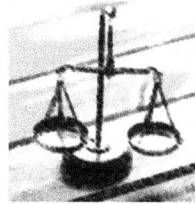

Likewise, Balance and Center are two closely related principles. In doing our tai chi form, Balance must be attained without leaning away from the Center. Balance allows fluid movement from one position to the next. The tai chi form should be done without a lot of up and down movement and often the optimum balance point for the limbs is at a forty-five (45°) degree angle or multiple thereof.

147

When discussing the concept of Balance concerning tai chi practice most people do not realize that this principle has several components. Or, perhaps they have just not given sufficient thought to the various aspects of this idea. In this section, I will present six different ways to think about the principle of "Balance".

• *Approach #1*: At the first and most basic level, there is simple physical balance (equilibrioception), the ability of the body to remain upright in the face of gravity. This is the one concept everyone immediately understands. It is this physical ability that we use for remaining upright when standing or walking or riding a bicycle or maneuvering a skateboard for example. It is both a state of bodily equilibrium and the ability to maintain that state. Physical balance results from and usually depends upon different bodily systems working harmoniously together. The eyes (visual system), ears (vestibular system), and the body's sense of where it is in space (proprioception) all contribute to our ability to maintain our balance. When these systems are intact and functioning properly good balance results automatically; no further conscious intervention is required.

• *Approach #2*: Balance has also been described as the opposition of equal forces. A state in which two opposing forces or factors are of equal strength or importance so that they effectively cancel each other out and stability is maintained. This second type of balance is certainly associated with tai chi, this idea of providing an equal response to a given stimulus. In a sense, it is related to cause and effect. Although equal and opposite forces are involved, I don't mean that you should respond to incoming physical force with a display of comparable physical force. That is not tai chi. That is a strength contest which the stronger person will surely win, all other things being equal. A better example is the simple action needed to jump up high. To do this, you first need to bend low and then spring up from the ground. The deeper you bend and flex the legs and the harder and more forcefully your legs push against the earth the higher you will go. Likewise, when you play drum and hit it hard you produce more sound; hit it with less force and you produce less sound.

148

Similarly, when you bounce a basketball on the floor the height of its rebound is directly dependent upon the force of its impact on the floor. The speed and force of the initial downward bounce will determine the speed and height of the resultant upward return bounce. Interestingly, when the ball is simply resting on the floor it rests at one point, its center point. When it is bounced on the floor it first hits at that one central point and then rebounds from that one central point. So, the center point is a related principle.

In tai chi as an applied martial art, you do not need to aggressively "defend" yourself. This statement sounds absurd until you understand that it is related to the idea of exhibiting an equal and balanced response in both your form and your partner work. Instead of learning how to launch a violent and forceful counter-attack, you train yourself to respond to the physical force exerted by the other person in a "soft overcomes hard manner". Other martial arts use force, strength, and speed to attack their opponent. In tai chi, we do not proceed in this manner. The paradox inherent in tai chi is that although it is done softly it is not weak.

Most people and many martial artists cannot understand this idea. They readily dismiss tai chi as being weak, ineffective, or hopelessly inadequate as a martial art. Yet the truth is that there is a balance here too. The degree of softness that is cultivated in tai chi practice is equal to the degree of hardness encountered in a martial arts opponent. It is just the opposite side of the coin. The two forces are equivalent and thus balanced. In tai chi, you are soft like water but this also enables you to be hard as steel. These two attributes are concurrent and equally present within the form and are utilized in tai chi as an applied martial art. The tai chi form is the physical expression of the Taoist idea of the simultaneous union and harmonized expression of the two distinct opposites depicted in the Yin-Yang symbol.

• *Approach #3:* A third way to think about balance concerns partner practice and how to respond to an attack in a manner that induces a state of imbalance in your partner. As I often tell my students, "Without Center, there can be no Balance. Without Balance, there can be no power". In tai chi, the idea of balance also includes the idea of not resisting the incoming force. You instead remain relaxed and yield in a timely manner so the incoming force has nowhere to land. Your partner encounters only emptiness in place of expected resistance and their power becomes harmlessly dispersed and neutralized. This in turn results in the partner losing both his or her Center and Balance while you retain yours.

"No Center, No Balance.
No Balance, No Power."

• *Approach #4:* The principle of Balance is also related to considerations of the Tao and the universal energy present in the tai chi form. I consider it essential that tai chi philosophy, tai chi form practice, and tai chi as a practical means of self-defense should all reflect a consistent point of view. If the theory and the practices do not coincide then there must be a defect in one or both aspects of the art. Based on over forty-five years of study and experience, I believe that traditional instruction should be reconsidered and revised.

As mentioned elsewhere, to resolve one such inconsistency, I believe changes are necessary regarding weight distribution in the legs. When standing in the Archer's Stance (bow stance), traditional tai chi instruction has the body's weight distributed 70% on the front foot and 30% on the rear foot. Unfortunately, such a postural position does not comply with Taoist philosophy regarding the union and interaction of forces that are equal and opposite, balanced and complementary.

To achieve such a corresponding result in tai chi form practice, I advocate and teach that when a person is positioned in the Archer's Stance the body's weight should instead be distributed 50% on the front foot and 50% on the back foot. Having the weight distributed in this manner creates Balance, maintains Center, and enables the connection of the Yin and Yang energy in the body. Of course, during certain form transitions from one posture to another, it is acceptable and often necessary to momentarily have 100% of the body's weight positioned over the "bubbling well" point of one foot or the other. However, as such transitions continue to the new posture, I tell my students to just return to the 50/50 weight distribution and to stop there. They are instructed and cautioned not to continue beyond this 50/50 position.

Whenever I have advanced this idea to other tai chi schools or another tai chi teacher, they immediately object to it. Their main criticism is that the 50/50 weight distribution in the feet creates a "double-weighted" condition in the body, a condition that tai chi practitioners must completely avoid. According to traditional thinking, a person who is "double-weighted" is considered to be out of balance and easier to defeat because he or she is not using the "cross substantial" energy inherent in the form. The "double-weighted" person is acting improperly by using just one side of the body to "defend/counterattack" the opponent. An example of such a "double-weighted" error would be having the weight in the forward, right foot while using just the right hand to perform some technique without any use of the left side of the body in the process.

I certainly agree that it is correct to say that in tai chi we must avoid a "double weighted" condition. However, that situation simply does not occur as a result of the 50/50 weight distribution in the feet which I advocate. This 50/50 placement of the body's position is not a "double-weighted" state. Instead, it allows the body to continuously remain in the Center of the "Globe Shape" and retain its Balance throughout the transitions from one posture to the next.

Having the weight distributed equally on the feet enables the upper body to be relaxed and light (*Yin*) while the lower body is solid and well-grounded through the rooted feet (*Yang*); thus, the body is in a true state of balance. If you stand with your weight distributed 70/30, your body is positioned too far forward and you are no longer Centered. If you are not Centered you can never achieve Balance. Being in your Center and maintaining that Center necessarily precedes your ability to attain a state of Balance.

Although the body may be relatively stable and upright in a 70/30 stance, it is in effect leaning and lacks a Center. Moving from one 70/30 stance to the next 70/30 stance necessitates that you momentarily dismantle your Center as you move the body to its next posture. Once in the new 70/30 position, then you must take additional time and effort to rebuild your Center to reestablish your Balance in the new posture. This type of change is not correct and is unnecessary. Additionally, if you lack Balance, it is also very difficult to get the "Globe Shape" that one should have and maintain throughout an entire round of form practice.

A major benefit of having the body's weight being distributed 50/50 in the feet and turning the Center before you shift to the new posture is that this allows you to maintain both your Center and your Balance at all times.

As I've mentioned elsewhere, the Taoist idea would be that the body is divided down the center. Front to back, side to side, top to bottom those divisions intersect at one Center point which is located at the core of the "Globe Shape". The division of the body in this manner results in a harmonious whole. The Yin and Yang become connected and equal; and, in turn, this unification results in an emergent property, the generation of chi.

In time, the cultivation of the body's chi energy which is developed during form practice will also beneficially enhance a person's sensitivity to and appreciation of both the positive and negative energy present in a broad variety of circumstances. There will be a heightened awareness of the type of chi associated with various people, or works of art, or the feng shui (a sense of the presence or absence of harmonious surroundings) in a particular place or location. This capability has allowed me to immediately sense and respond when there is any unease or imbalance in a given situation. For example, during a routine shopping excursion with a student, I unexpectedly came upon a severe energetic imbalance surrounding certain artifacts in the store. (See Appendix "E", At the Antique Store.)

• *Approach #5*: There is also a fifth way to think about balance. In your partner practice, and most certainly in uncooperative/competitive practice, you must realize that a loss is not a defeat or failure. It involves something more than just losing. Such partner practice is not just a one-sided, zero-sum, the winner takes all event. When you lose you are also gaining something of equal value, experience. Hence, there is much wisdom in the instruction to "invest in loss" as part of your tai chi training.

It has long been said in tai chi that you must "invest in loss" or "eat bitter". If you invest in loss you will increase in everything. Rather than "investment in loss" I prefer the phrase "acceptance of loss" because this implies that you are willing to not allow your ego to get in the way of your training. The training method should encourage your partner to push you. If you learn to "accept" the push you will increase your leg strength, foot strength, and root. In time, where you thought there was no available space to yield effectively, your body will find more space in which to respond and neutralize the incoming force. You become better able to avoid the push or punch. In a fight situation, you will have attained a fast reaction time and good balance.

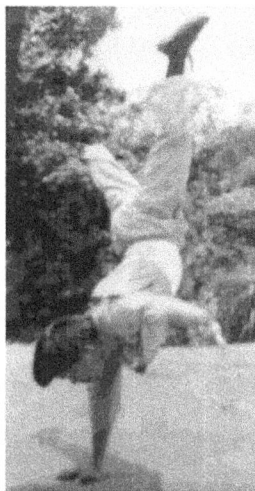

Handstand, Master Wang

While each person is positioned opposite the other in the Archer's Stance, I will train students by first decreasing the distance between them significantly. Then I have the pusher place his or her front foot lightly on top of the partner's rearfoot and pin it to the floor. This makes it very difficult to yield and respond to the incoming push in a soft and neutralizing manner but it is very worthwhile training in "eating bitter" and "accepting loss".

I know from my experience in tai chi Push Hands competitions that success is often achieved through the use of clever techniques and certain effective patterns of movement. When engaged in uncooperative/competitive practice, the preferable and superior objective should instead be to deal with the situation in a relaxed and soft manner. You should seek to neutralize the opponent's incoming force and then allow it to return to the opponent. The quality you want to cultivate is one of extreme softness. In learning to do this you will certainly be unsuccessful many, many times; but, from my experience, I can tell you that with each loss your abilities will improve. Given enough time and practice, this extremely soft method becomes extremely powerful. Most people probably do not believe that to be the case but I have found that it is true and attainable. Things will balance out.

• *Approach #6:* There is a sixth way to think about balance. Tai chi's balance principle can be a metaphor for life. To lead a successful life, you need to keep all aspects well-balanced.

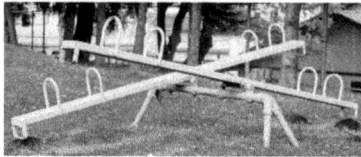

◆ ◆ ◆

移動全動

Coordination

7th Principle: Coordination

In dictionaries, you will find that Coordination (Whole Body Unification) is defined as the skillful and balanced movement of different parts, especially parts of the body, at the same time. It can include the combining of diverse parts or groups to make a unit or the way these parts work together in unison. Harmonization, organization, management, synchronization are all related terms.

In our daily lives, when we go out for a walk our bodies are naturally coordinated. When one's left leg moves forward, one's right arm balances it. There is no hesitation or separation of movement among the body's parts. They are simply synchronized.

Coordination

Similarly, for Coordination to occur in the tai chi form there can be no separation of movement. The upper and lower body must move in unison, the left side must balance the right. When one's arms are raised the knees descend. When pressure is applied to the right leg, the left arm compensates. Just as in walking, the movements in the form must be synchronized in time and space and the body must move as a unit.

One of the reasons that I place Coordination as the final attribute on the Seven Principles list is that it is usually the last element to be perfected in one's tai chi form practice. It seems to take the longest to appear. Perhaps this is because the form requires us to make various unfamiliar shapes and assume various unaccustomed postures. We take on ways of moving our bodies that we don't otherwise regularly encounter in our daily lives. So too, both Push Hands and "Search Center" play put us in situations in which our bodies and minds are faced with many novel experiences. Experiences that are constantly changing and that can come and go so rapidly that we can be left wondering, "what just happened?" Consequently, partner practice, particularly uncooperative/competitive partner practice, offers a unique challenge to the maintenance of proper coordination.

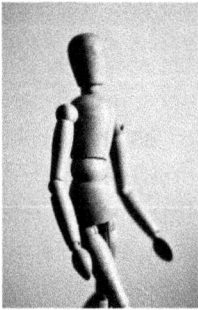

For Coordination to develop the body needs lots of repetitive form practice. Achieving Coordination is dependent upon such practice. When first learning the form every move that is made seems very complicated and the timing of the movements is incorrect. Eventually one makes the transition from feeling that form practice is complex to find it very simple. Your chi, your form, your body, and your mind become integrated. The distinct parts of the body have become organized and interconnected in a new way. You realize that all movements in the form are only one type of movement. That is, they all have the same inherent qualities present while being performed. A sort of "sixth sense" develops and when the body is in motion the form postures become one unified state of being.

• *The Results of Principle-Based Practice:* As a result of our tai chi form practice, we get more chi flowing in our body and our health is improved. The body also behaves more naturally and we become less awkward in our movements. The overall suppleness and flexibility of the body are increased as well. These results are the effect of coordination on the physical level. But as an outcome of our tai chi practice, we also become more coordinated on the spiritual level. We are less "strangers" to ourselves and more comfortable in our being. We are better able to cope with life's ever-changing circumstances and become more harmonious in our relationships with other people. We become more like water. Water can adapt so that it fits any container in which it is placed. We develop a fuller understanding of life and it becomes happier, more stable, and well-balanced.

I need to pause here to remind you of another essential idea. Although I have been discussing various attributes associated with each of my individual Seven Principles, it is important to realize and remember that all these principles apply equally and simultaneously to your tai chi form practice. They are intertwined and mutually reinforcing. It is through the combination and integration of all seven of them at the same time that your tai chi practice will improve.

It is also important to mention here that the various stages in the development of one's tai chi practice must occur one after the other. There are no shortcuts. A person must devote himself or herself to progressing through each stage. You can't just leap to the end.

Once the Seven Principles are integrated into your practice, doing the tai chi form will become more and more a "moving meditation". Performing just one posture can include and contain everything you've studied and that posture becomes full of the soft power which results from the cultivation of the internal chi. At this stage, the formation of postural shapes and the various patterns of movement are no longer a major concern. Your Yi and Chi are well developed and you are working at the Shen level. This is a later, more advanced stage of your tai chi development. However, only a few people can attain this Shen stage as it requires countless hours of disciplined practice and for most tai chi players their days are too busy with the other demands of daily life.

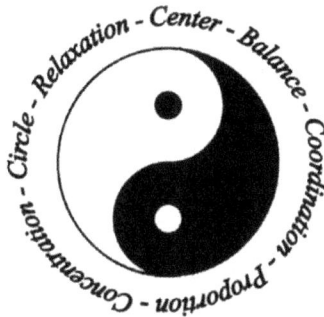

"Yong Yi, Bu Yong Li."

"Use the mind, not force."

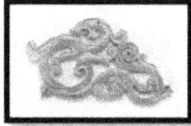

Chapter 10: Rules for Tai Chi Form Practice

OVER HUNDREDS OF years, the Chinese developed a remarkable variety of hard-style and soft-style martial arts systems. Many of the form postures found in those systems have common characteristics and even share a common origin. Their source can be traced back to early Taoist practices. Those practices were initially created and cultivated as a means to promote health and longevity. They were not necessarily constructed for purposes of combat or self-defense. This is particularly true regarding the origins of the postures found in the various styles of tai chi.

• *Following Nature's Way:* The early Taoists made a special point of watching how a diverse assortment of creatures behaved in nature. They closely studied the habits and routines of various animals, birds, fish, insects, and reptiles. As a result, they became adept at cataloging the movements which were most characteristic of numerous species. From those behavioral observations, the Taoists then developed health-promoting calisthenics which mimicked the wide range of nature's activities they had seen. Sets of exercises were constructed based upon a variety of animal-related themes. For example, the crane, the bear, the monkey, the deer, and the snake were all used as inspirations for the form and content of an assortment of physical exercises. Many of the movements copied the activities performed by the creature being imitated. It was thought that by following the laws of nature rather than acting in opposition to them, people would become aligned with the natural order of things. Thereby, their health would be strengthened and harmony with the natural world could be realized.

• *Various Styles of Tai Chi:* An array of different styles of tai chi forms have developed over the years. One common element among them is that each seeks to create a connection between the development of internal power and its manifestation in external movement. In doing so, they each follow, to one degree or another, that same Taoist viewpoint regarding the need to align one's actions by following nature and the natural world and to not act in opposition to it.

Today, perhaps the best known and most widely practiced major forms of tai chi are the Chen, Yang, Wu/Hao, Wu, and Sun forms. Historically the Chen style was the original of these five forms and the rest followed. The order I've given here is the generally accepted sequence of their chronological development. Each form arose more or less from the one which preceded it. Of these five, the Yang Style is probably the one most widely known and practiced, at least in the West. The Chen Style is the next most well-known style. The Sun, Wu, and Hao forms are not as well-known nor as widely practiced in the West.

Each of these five styles of tai chi contains a series of distinct postures that are practiced in a customary sequence. Although the number of postures contained in each form may vary, the student of any one of these styles would certainly recognize many, if not most, of the postures from any of the other styles. Although each style shares a large number of common postures, the way a particular posture is performed in each of the different styles can vary in many significant respects. For example, the instructions for the posture "Brush Knee" (or substitute almost any other posture name here) as taught in the Yang Style are not the same as those in the Chen Style. So too, the sequence of the postures and the actions taken while transitioning from one posture to the next are not always the same. Nor are the completed positions that constitute the full posture identical. For example, the posture "Single Whip" when performed in the Wu Style resembles that of the Yang Style but the position of the feet and the orientation of the trunk and waist are completely different. So, each style has developed a different pathway in the presentation of its various form postures.

At the risk of oversimplification in making my point, I would characterize the movements and postures of the Yang Style form as being relaxed and smooth. Those of the Chen Style, and to a certain extent the Wu Style as well, place more emphasis on spiraling movements and the development of demonstrable power. Those of the Sun Style and Hao Style take yet another direction. Their styles consist of smaller outward movements while developing a more internal use of energy.

The very existence and longevity of these various tai chi styles is certainly an indication that they each must have considerable merit. Each has millions of practitioners around the world and each has produced a number of writings, instructions, and notably accomplished teachers. However, this rather extensive variety of instructions, presentations, cautions, and advice can be quite confusing to any beginning student who seeks to learn the art of tai chi. The beginner has no frame of reference from which to decide who is right. Can they all be right? Which is the "best" one to study?

Before moving to North America, I had not had much exposure to the Western staple grain, wheat. I soon learned that it was grown to make flour which in turn people used to make dough. That basic dough enabled them to make all kinds of bread, cakes, pastries, and the bakery's many other delicious temptations. But all these nourishing and enjoyable items start with a dough made from simple flour. That dough is then formed into different patterns and each pattern is given a particular name. This is a bagel, that is a doughnut.

This dough analogy is similar to what occurs in tai chi. The internal chi is like flour which is made into a dough. The different styles of tai chi are like the different baked goods which can be made from the same dough mixture. We take the dough of internal chi power and use the different forms of tai chi to create the external expression of the internal energy. The postures in the form are like the finished goods in the bakery's display case. Faithful, daily practice of the form is where it all starts; it sows the seeds that grow and nourish that internal chi.

To me, the external postural differences which are evident in these various tai chi styles are not the issue. Moreover, they should not be the basis for any disputes between the practitioners of one style versus another. Whether you practice Chen Style, Yang Style or yet some other style is not what is important. The important point is whether, as a result of your practice, you have been able to develop your chi and enhance your health. For me, the fundamental reason we undertake the practice of any tai chi form, regardless of the particular style, is to use that form to create and strengthen our internal chi energy. In so doing, we will be more likely to enjoy a long, healthy, and harmonious life.

• *The Four Qualities of All Form Practice:* No matter which style you choose to study, there should be four qualities evident in your form practice, namely: (1.) Relaxation, (2.) Center, (3.) Openness, and (4.) Softness.

Relaxation and Center are two of my Seven Principles. The characteristic elements associated with each of these qualities are discussed in Chapter 9.

• *Open the Mind:* By "openness" I mean open your body of course but I also mean open your mind to new ways of thinking. The

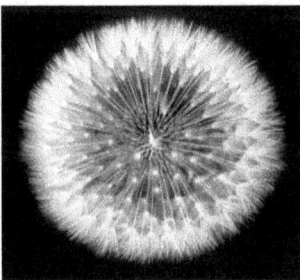

mind teaches the body. The body listens to the mind's instructions. When the mind commands, the body follows even down to the cellular level. The mind's influence is capable of changing each cell in the body. During this process, there is also a certain relationship to universal energy which is found everywhere in the natural world. The body's cells connect to the universal energy and become more unified. They also transfer the information of the universal energy to the body itself. The entire body in turn becomes more unified as its cells connect to universal energy.

• *Disunity in Form Practice:*   Stringing together a precisely composed and accurate series of form postures is surely the best way to facilitate the accumulation and flow of the internal energy. Unfortunately, when most people practice their tai chi form their movements are usually done incorrectly. Although well-intentioned, their practice is incorrect in the sense that it lacks all the requisite components needed for constructing proper form. The initial and most common error is a physical one. Their execution of the form is incomplete because the parts of the body are not yet consistently connected and unified in a well-coordinated manner. Also, the requisite union of the body and the mind/intent (*Yi*) has not been fully achieved either. Those two required yet elusive unifications must be made.

Form practice can be likened to making fire with a flint. At first, you strike the rock repeatedly without success. Suddenly you get an isolated spark and are encouraged to keep trying. Then you try again and again to make another spark, and another spark, and another spark until in the end you light the fire. Many attempts and many failures will be required but eventually, all that hard work, that kung fu, will lead to success if people conduct their tai chi form practice according to the proper principles, principles found in nature.

When a breakthrough in form practice occurs, it is like finding the key to deciphering an encrypted message. Without the key, no one can comprehend it. With the key, the message can be understood. Eventually, almost as if by accident, that breakthrough will occur and a practitioner will catch the right idea and the correct sensation/feeling while doing the form. They will have found their key. Then the task of their practice is to try to recapture and reproduce that sensation/feeling consistently thereafter throughout the entire form and in all the transitions from posture to posture. This is what I call being on the tai chi trail, a concept that is discussed in greater detail elsewhere in this book. The more times that a practitioner undertakes form practice of a mindful and principle-based nature the more their tai chi form will all come together until one day it will be right. (See Chapter 12, "Transitions & the Chi Trail".)

• *Tai Chi as a Meditation Art:* It was only after I had been practicing tai chi for about ten years that I began a deeper study in an attempt to truly understand what the tai chi form was all about.

Tai chi form practice is like a meditation exercise. Indeed, many before me have called it a moving meditation. In many forms of seated meditation practice, the student is given a single, specific phrase to repeat or a simple task to perform to assist the quieting and focusing of the mind. Counting the breath, gazing at a candle, or reciting a mantra are some commonly used devices. The mind is given something for the imagination to fix on which, with sufficient practice, will enable the student to quiet the mind and find a path to a more internal state of being. Tai chi form practice can be likened to meditation in that respect. It can lead to a highly focused and more advanced internal mental state of being.

The central idea behind tai chi as a moving meditation is that of cultivating a deeply felt state of relaxation *(Sung)*. The student seeks to root, allow the energy to sink, catch his or her balance, and find the proper proportional relationships of the limbs and trunk as required by the various postures of the form. If the student is not thinking about fighting or the applied martial arts aspects of the postures, his or her form will become softer and float along effortlessly while still being properly rooted. This will allow the chi to circulate more readily.

If instead, as is now commonly taught, you are thinking about how to use this particular series of shapes or patterns in the form as part of a martial arts system, a different idea and mindset are in operation. It is a mindset assigned to conflict and contention. Such a mindset is not conducive to the cultivation of a relaxed state of being in both mind and body. If you think that way, you are already trapped, already using strength, and already entangled in fighting, whether you consciously realize it or not. Practicing your tai chi form using this combative method of thought will not lead to either relaxation or smoothness in your form. It can result in the opposite.

Since achieving and maintaining a deeply relaxed state is essential to the development and cultivation of internal chi, any training which doesn't foster it is not very useful or beneficial. The student should not be thinking about how to use a particular posture as a martial arts application. The imagery to be used should not be downgraded to that of confrontation and fighting. The imagery should instead be any imagery that cultivates a sense of calm, peacefulness, and relaxation. When you think in this way you will feel more confident. Your insides will feel looser and smoother. This in turn will help create internal chi.

In some respects, there is little that looks like actual fighting in the tai chi form. Perhaps you did not realize this. For example, in all tai chi movements, the palms remain open. Even when forming a punch, the hands don't close into the clenched fist that is commonly associated with Western-style boxing. In the tai chi punch, the fingers are held loosely not firmly and the fist is open in the middle not closed. Although the pads of the fingertips touch the palm, the contact they make is extremely light and a slight hollow is maintained as if holding a raw egg or fluffy caterpillar.

Most people today are thinking about and practicing the tai chi form in a manner related to its perceived martial arts applications. In practicing with this mindset their tai chi form can take on an undesirable hardness. When that happens the circulation of the chi energy becomes blocked and it will not flow as readily or even at all. Their chi becomes stuck.

To use ideas related to the fighting arts is to use the wrong images. Particularly in the early stages, the time when you are starting on the path of developing your internal energy, the use of fighting imagery is unquestionably counterproductive. In the absence of the development and flow of internal energy, the premature focus on the martial arts aspects of the form is like putting the cart before the horse. The martial arts applications contained in the postures will lack the prerequisite internal energy which is the true hallmark and distinguishing characteristic of the art. This may sound harsh perhaps but my experience tells me it is an accurate description of the outcome for far too many long-time practitioners.

There is little or no use of internal energy evident in their partner interactions.

There is an expression that describes tai chi form as "long fist" or as "long boxing". By this, it is meant that it is similar to a river on which the tai chi player floats along. It has no beginning and no end. It simply flows while the tai chi player's actions are smooth, even, relaxed, and proceed unceasingly. This state of being is not easy to achieve in doing one's tai chi form. It can easily take five years of regular, daily practice before one begins to achieve it. Yet, this is what the art requires.

The methods and mindsets used in the traditional manner of teaching tai chi can seem practically counterproductive to the development and use of one's internal chi. On the one hand, while you practice the solo form, you are advised to visualize an opponent in front of you and that you are utilizing each posture in a marital application to overcome and defeat him or her. On the other hand, when faced with a real opponent in Push Hands practice or a competitive Push Hands tournament, you are advised to practice your form movements as if no one is standing in front of you. I maintain that you are better able to develop internal chi during form practice if you do not think about the martial applications at all since this will encourage the deeper relaxation of both body and mind. During partner practice of any type, I emphasize that you should focus your complete attention and listening skills (*ting jin*) on your partner instead of imagining they are not present.

Of course, everyone realizes that tai chi is indeed a martial art. The literal English translation can be "Supreme Ultimate Fist" or "Supreme Ultimate Boxing" or some such equivalent. It certainly can be highly effective when used in that manner by a skilled practitioner. My point here is not to deny that tai chi is a formidable martial art. The point I do want to make is perhaps a subtler one concerning the imagery associated with the name of this art. Its very name denotes fighting and thus, in some respects, breaks the image of peaceful harmony which is said to underlie and be the authentic tai chi way. Based on my years of experience, I have concluded that to better develop the internal energy component of the art tai chi teachers should give their students images that lack the element of fighting or the use of external physical force.

To achieve consistency between theory and practice, I developed my Seven Principles. These principles apply at all times, whether practicing the form or participating in partner work, whether Push Hands or "Search Center". There is no inconsistency or conflict when engaged in either of those two aspects of tai chi practice. These principles are also universal and readily apply to every style of tai chi. Ranked in order of importance they are: (1.) Relaxation, (2.) Center, (3.) Concentration, (4.) Circle, (5.) Proportion, (6.) Balance, and (7.) Coordination. (See Chapter 9, "The Seven Principles of Tai Chi".).

◆ ◆ ◆

Some Observations on the Practice of Tai Chi Form:

Regardless of the chosen style, the first level in anyone's tai chi practice is simply to learn the pattern and sequences of movements that constitute the postures of that style. It is perhaps equivalent to learning the scales and chords in music. When you are learning to play a musical instrument, the more time you devote to practice the better you become at controlling that instrument. Control in turn enables you to better capture the underlying feeling of the music. The interpretive flow of the composition can then be better expressed. Similarly, in tai chi, the more you practice the form, the more you gain control over your body; and, the more you can unify the mind and the body. As this ability develops, you will begin to feel the flow of the chi just as the musician feels the flow of the piece he or she is playing. The following observations may be useful to your form practice.

• *Stand Up. Don't Let the Knees Bend Too Low:* One of my Seven Principles for form practice is the requirement to maintain your own Center. This concept is not limited to just dividing your body in half whether front to back, side to side, top and bottom. It also involves the proper development of the root from the top of the head, through your spine, and down into the foot and earth. Having a sound root allows the various joints and parts of the body to act as one so that the whole body can move as one unit. Of course, the mind should be focused and connected to the body's unified movement as well.

Frequently, teachers will instruct students to sink into their roots. Many students and some teachers are under the mistaken impression that to sink properly they should drop their bodies lower by bending the knees at an unduly deep angle. Although the knees are indeed slightly bent and certainly not locked during tai chi practice, this bending at the knees can be overdone. When this happens, the physical body cannot handle the unnecessary, excessive pressure; and, this causes blockage of the chi flow and disruption of a true rooted connection to the ground.

There is a difference between muscle system training and training to open the chi flow. In this context, the sinking into one's root involves not so much the physical act of taking a lower stance. Instead, it is more properly associated with an internal sensation of the release of unnecessary muscular tension throughout the body such that the upper body's hardness and stiffness are drained to the point where it feels light (*Yin*) while the lower body becomes more stable (*Yang*) in its connection to the earth. When the chi is accumulated in the lower dan tien and the body is *Sung*, harnessing the earth's Yin energy and combining it with heaven's Yang energy will encourage the inner chi to develop and flow.

In tai chi, it is not necessary to train the muscles by taking what I would call an extremely low stance. Doing so can make it harder to develop your internal chi power. The traditional rule that the knee of the forward leg should be aligned with the foot and never extend forward beyond the toes is correct. However, there should be a related rule which states that it is unnecessary to adopt a very low stance even if the knee does not go beyond the toe. Instead of taking an extremely low stance, if you stand taller and keep your weight distributed 50/50 on the feet you become properly centered and you will have a better root.

• *Reconsidering Tai Chi Imagery:* I am interested in the development of a new approach to form practice. My training method is different from the traditional martial arts way. To develop internal chi power, I believe that the student will benefit from having appropriate images for the mind to latch onto. Of particular importance is that such imagery promotes and helps generate a sense of calmness, relaxation, tranquility, and peacefulness. When you think in this way you will feel more confident. Your insides will feel looser and smoother. This in turn will help create internal chi.

I have concluded that the images used while doing the tai chi form need to be changed from those associated with fighting an opponent to those associated with a more calm and relaxed state of being. By choosing these more serene images the mind and body are better able to relax and thus the chi can grow and flow more productively.

For example, there is a well-known group of four successive postures, Ward Off (*Peng*), Rollback (*Lu*), Press (*Ji*), and Push (*An*) which are collectively known as the "Grasp Sparrows Tail" sequence. The origin of this colorful description can be found in the ancient practice of falconry in which birds of prey, such as hawks and falcons, were kept as pets and taught to hunt on command. When not aloft, the birds perch on the falconer's forearm where they are often stroked and petted by their handlers. It is this imagery of gently stroking the bird's tail which is the more suitable imagery to be used when practicing that portion of the form by yourself; and, even more so when engaged with your partner in the two-person training exercise in which those four postures are featured.

When I teach the tai chi form, I do not recite the names of the various postures, either in Chinese or the customary English translations. Nor do I use words that invoke fighting imagery or words that describe the applied martial arts function contained in each pose. Instead, I just tell my students, "Okay, here is the next tai chi shape." In doing so, I am consciously seeking a way to change the imagery associated with the form so that it is not related to fighting. The reason I teach the form in this way is that I want to align a student's form-related imagery with the underlying tai chi philosophy of seeking softness and relaxation in one's movements.

171

I would encourage you to do the same in your practice. Don't think about "Brush Knee" as an action that can in part redirect and neutralize the opponent's kick while simultaneously delivering a blow. Don't think about the "Deflect, Parry, and Punch" movements as having a martial arts application. Instead, think about it as just chopping wood. Use the weight and momentum of the ax in your hands; let it fall without added effort and let nature's force of gravity split the wood. Another example would be "Low Punch". Do not think punch; instead, perhaps think of playing lawn bowls or bocce ball.

What you want to achieve when performing those three postures, or any other posture, is a spiral rotation of the internal line of energy. That's all. If instead, you are thinking about striking an opponent you are focusing on the wrong thing. You are sabotaging your ability to recognize and cultivate the correct sensations associated with the presence and flow of that spiraling line of internal energy as it manifests in each different posture. This manifestation of the internal energy (*nei jin*) will be exhibited somewhat differently in each posture; and, you need to understand how that occurs and what it feels like.

In my tai chi journey, I have had at least ten different teachers. Each of them was highly skilled and I respected and learned a great deal from them all. But, as I have mentioned previously, each of them had a different approach to tai chi form practice. For example, when doing the "Push" (*An*) posture I was variously taught to use hand power, and then short power, or then to act in a manner that was more like Shaolin boxing. But in subsequent years I instead realized that the image best suited to the cultivation of chi energy when doing the "Push" posture is that of simply propelling a boat from a standing position while using a single oar. Similar to a Venetian gondolier, each time you move forward and back you seek to smoothly put the oar in the water and gently glide the boat across the calm waters.

One of my students told me that he occasionally substitutes another gentle image when teaching the "Press (*Ji*) to Push (*An*)" transition in his classes. As the students transfer out of "Press" to the rear foot they are instructed to open their hands and "catch the baby in the swing"; and, as they move forward, to gently "push the baby in the swing".

Tai chi form practice should be peaceful, undisturbed, and without interruption. The correct imagery and way of thinking should be calm and composed. Don't think of the tai chi form as having a particular function or any martial arts applications at all. Think instead that it is useless. Think of it as dancing with the chi. When you practice the form, focus instead on becoming the person who understands and exemplifies the Seven Principles. Using such an indirect approach can be said to follow Lao Tse's philosophy to arrive at one's intended destination. It is just another of the many paradoxes inherent in tai chi.

• *Turn the Center First, Then Shift the Weight:* To my way of thinking traditional tai chi instruction has, quite unintentionally, lead to the development of many problems that stand in the way of a student's development of their optimum chi potential. For example, when changing from one posture to the next, the traditional common directive is to first shift the weight and then turn the Center in the direction of the new posture. This way of moving between postures is not the best possible way to move if one seeks to develop internal power.

Let me be clear about this point, it is not that you can never develop internal power if you first shift the weight and then turn the body. Certainly, there have been accomplished masters who have developed such energy by using that method. What I am suggesting is that this is not the optimum way to move.

Instead, my perhaps controversial proposition is that when moving from one posture to the next you should first turn your Center and only then shift the weight. I maintain that this is the optimum way to transition between any two postures. I realize that this is contrary to what others have said. Nevertheless, my experience tells me that is the better way to develop your internal power.

Why? The answer is that the Center is the leader of the body's weight and the pivot point around which our bodies revolve. Here I mean the term "Center" to include the vertical axis of the body as well as the point where that axis meets and crosses the horizontal axis of the body; this is also the lower dan tien area which is the location of the center of gravity for our bodies. When the Center turns first the movement of the rest of your body must automatically follow that rotation. From the head to the spine and on down through the entire body to the foot, once the Center turns, the entire body also turns.

"Turn the Center First, Then Shift the Weight."

When doing your form, you should keep your mind on maintaining the Center. From your head, through your spine, down to your lower dan tien, and then down to your foot, this is the line of the Center. You never allow your body to lean to one side. If you lean, the Center is divided and your well-balanced position is compromised.

Before you can begin to make a turn of the waist (here I mean pelvis and hips) you first need to catch the centerline. By consciously catching the centerline, you become aware of your center point and are then able to move circularly around it, just like a spinning coin or toy top. This centerline axis of the head, waist, and foot all follow the line of balance which gravity provides to connect the whole body as a unit. Ballerinas when turning on point and figure skaters when executing a high-speed spin are examples of this rotational principle. In this method, you also do not allow the head to turn independently. You should turn your Center first and then shift the weight. Turn, then transfer your movement into the next posture. (See Chapter 11, "Three Keys to Tai Chi Form" for a discussion regarding the position of the head.)

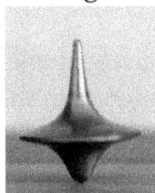

This is a very important and significant idea. You first turn, then shift. Having this centerline established and turning on the related

174

axis is a major part of my method for developing internal energy. If you move your body in the way I suggest, you can use this axis to create the internal spiral power. Otherwise, if you shift the weight first and then turn, you will never get the center spiral occurring inside your body. By turning first, you are keeping the body on that central spiral all the time. Having stayed on that central spiral you can then shift into the next posture and you'll never lose the center pole. (See also Chapter 9, the 2nd Principle: Center)

This is different from a similar Chi Kung exercise which also repeatedly turns back and forth, left to right, or right to left. That Chi Kung exercise does not develop the internal spiral that we seek to train in our tai chi form.

• *Developing the Internal Spiral:* The energy line being developed by moving this way is not like the energy used in training the "Pull" (*Tsai*) or "Push" (*An*) postures. Instead, it involves how to train the origination of motion from your Center. When your Center develops this spiraling, spring-like coil you can use the stored energy which results from its compression and release. There is no external movement. You can feel that the coil inside is being squeezed and that the resultant internal power comes from there. The power does not come from just your hand pushing back; it comes from your Center and the entire, unified body.

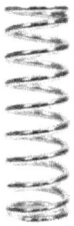

This central axis must first be related to your foot (your tai chi root). Then you transmit the energy taken from the ground to the waist (again, pelvis and hips). Then the turn of the waist brings the turn of the trunk. The result of this sequential type of movement is the creation of a spiral line which is initiated from the planted foot's relaxed attachment to the earth. The torque-like motion increases your internal spiral. The internal strength and power of the movement come from this internal energy line. The more you practice in this manner the more coordinated your actions will become. So, first, turn your Center. Then, shift your weight. That is an important aspect of my method.

• *The Arms Don't Lead, They Follow:* When doing the form, it is helpful to think of nature just as the old Taoist masters did. For example, think of watching a fish swim. Watch closely and you will see that the fish first moves from its center; the trunk leads and the tail follows. Thus, in doing your tai chi form the proper sequence of movement is that once having established the central axis from the foot's ground connection, the trunk leads, then the arm comes last to finish the movement. Just like a fish's tail is the last thing to move, so too the arm is the last to move when doing the form. "Let the trunk carry the arms.", I often say.

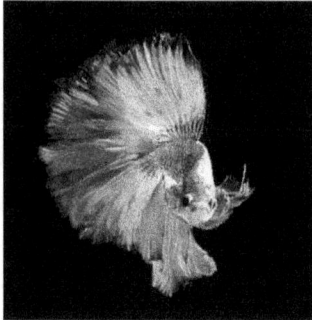

"Turn the Center First. Let the Trunk Carry the Arms."

Once the weight is transferred, then the arms follow. The key point here is that when doing your tai chi form the arm should never lead the movement. It does not and must not go first. Instead, the arm should follow your body as if gliding afterward. Also, the arm should not be performing a task; it has no purpose as it moves. You should not be thinking that the arm has to accomplish some martial arts assignment or achieve a result such as a punch or a block or a parry. Rather, it simply follows along as the trunk is turned and the weight is shifted. You most certainly should not be imagining, visualizing, or even be thinking about any martial arts application associated with the arm's position in any posture. Fight-related imagery is not conducive to the development of internal energy.

• *Opening the Joints:* In practicing the tai chi form, you are training to be able to do two things at once when you are engaged in partner practice. One is to take in or absorb the energy from your partner. The other is to return it. For example, I am capable of using my "Ward Off" (*Peng*) arm to support and hold off the incoming forces when two, three, or four people simultaneously push on it; and

176

then I can instantly discharge all of them at once so they "fly away" backward.

When training "Ward Off" (*Peng*), with one person or several pushing on your forearm, the first thing you need to do is make an energetic connection to your partner and simultaneously absorb his or her incoming pressure. To absorb and redirect that incoming energy, you need to open the joints of your body. Learning to open the joints in this way is what allows you to redirect the incoming force. If you are closed anywhere in your joints, no matter how much you may want that incoming energy to go down the center and be harmlessly dispersed into the ground, you will be unable to do that. If your joints are closed the interaction then becomes merely an exercise in physical strength, a contest to determine who is the stronger. (See Chapter 12, "Transitions & The Chi Trail".)

The ability to open the joints is directly related to the degree of whole-body relaxation (*Sung*) you have achieved as a result of your form practice. Among other things, when the form is practiced in a slow, deliberate, and intentional manner the nine joints become open. My students ask me how they will recognize the physical sensations in their bodies that tell them that they are open? I tell them it just takes lots of practice.

• *Relaxation & Interconnected Unity:* It is a mistake to think that the constant command to relax while doing your practice is a call to seek relaxation for its own sake. The basis for achieving the ability to be interconnected throughout the body is found in the relaxation you cultivate while doing the tai chi form. From the rooted foot each movement rises through the legs, the pelvis rotates via the hip joint or *kwa* (kua) area, the Center turns, and then the arms move last. To maintain this connection, the coordinated timing of the movements is essential. If the movement is instead segmented the spiral is lost and the chi does not flow freely. Relaxation allows us to achieve the ultimate goal of having the body's separate parts become interconnected and become one. I think understanding that point is what is important.

By "one" I mean that you can open all your joints and your Center so that there is one connection through your whole body from the top of the head to the ground. For example, imagine that you are using a two-handed Push (*An*) against my Ward Off (*Peng*) arm. To join into one, I let my body relax and align it with you. Then I funnel or squeeze everything associated with your incoming energy down to one point. Doing so allows me to absorb your incoming force.

After you have experienced and experimented with this Ward Off/Absorb the Push feeling many, many times you will develop what I call the "chi trail" in your partner work just as you have done in your form practice. You can imagine this trail and control it and then add your chi to it so it becomes powerful.

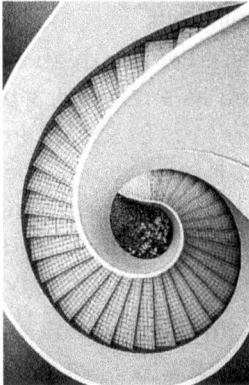

To absorb your partner's incoming energy, you first need to able to organize your own body so that it becomes one, becomes structurally unified in a relaxed (*Sung*) manner. This in turn will enable you to connect the joints of the body through to the ground. Having done so, you now have inside you that chi trail. It is like a coiled spring or spiraled pathway. By letting the relaxation evolve you will be able to discover this trail for yourself. But this takes time. As this evolution occurs, your body will become more capable and certain in managing its proper, coordinated response to the incoming force; and, at the same time, it will be more relaxed. The resultant relaxation and increased capabilities of this unified body allow your body to remain naturally calm and at ease. That's why relaxation is not sought just for its own sake. So that's a major point.

For a proper state of tai chi relaxation to be manifested, you want your body to become a fully integrated and cohesive unit. When the parts of the body are properly aligned and united, the rhythm of the movement coupled with the mind/intent (*Yi*) will allow the *nei jin* to produce a smooth transfer of power and energy through the structure. This integration is a distinct qualitative state which can be felt in the body. The experience of what such a unified bodily state feels like is not easy to accurately or adequately convey on the printed page. The assistance of an experienced teacher or accomplished practice partner is of great benefit in helping you reach and recognize the correct feeling. Particularly between practice partners, it is important to cooperate and have patience with each other as you each explore the various demands and potentials available in tai chi form work.

• *The Chi Trail:* Practicing your tai chi form builds this chi trail. When doing the form, this trail needs to be maintained at all times. It must be present in the full posture but it also must be preserved during each transitional moment from posture to posture. This continuous trail idea is related to the concept of the Circle in my Seven Principles. Each point on the transition between postures is like a degree on the circumference of a circle. For example, if you took a series of freeze-frame pictures, at each instant the connection must be present. No gaps should occur. You want to be able to find that trail consistently, again and again. Time after time. As you develop the trail it will bring energy and power. (See also Chapter 12, "Transitions & The Chi Trail".)

As you practice your form, do not make the mistake of thinking about the actual martial arts application of any posture. If you think that that there is some purpose or function behind doing a particular posture then you are already engaged at just the physical level and not the internal chi level. Thinking about the martial applications will cause you to lose the trail. You should think of the form as not having any useful purpose. By adopting this approach, you eliminate the applied martial arts mindset and that will allow you to focus instead on using the trail sensations as a connection method for the unification of the mind/intent (*Yi*) and the body.

While discussing partner work, one of my senior students said if he goes into the "Push" (*An*) posture thinking that he will use it to push someone out, as would happen in a Push Hands contest, the chi seems to disappear. He says that merely thinking of applying the martial application of the "Push" causes him to lose his own Center, lose connection within himself and that the related chi sensations immediately vanish.

His report echoes my point. It should not be your purpose to develop the physical power (*Li*) usually associated with the physical act of "pushing". From having that kind of purpose and thinking about achieving that "push" result, everything related to the internal energy stops, and the chi is gone. Why? The correct idea behind cultivating that internal energy is now gone. This is exactly what I am talking about concerning the "uselessness" of the tai chi form. This simple, illogical, and paradoxical idea will bring out the inherent power of the soft way.

• *Theory Should Precede Practice:* Much tai chi practice today is done without the participants having any understanding of the basic principles which underlie the movements. Moreover, they don't understand why tai chi is done slowly, they don't understand why tai chi seeks to move in a relaxed way, they don't understand why they are not standing in a low stance. What they need is a good theoretical foundation for their practice before they start doing tai chi form work.

If you start your tai chi studies with the idea that you will first copy the external movement pattern of the form and learn to work the internal energy aspects of form practice later, you are already working at cross purposes. In proceeding this way, you are not acting in your own best interest. Your external state and your mental state are totally in conflict. This means that you are still only working at just a physical level.

The reason for the slow tempo and relaxed manner is that to be able to do tai chi properly you must first try to give up your physical tension, be soft. Tai chi's deliberate and unhurried manner of movement requires good balance, flexibility, timing, and coordination which is why many beginners and even more experienced students find it awkward to do and more difficult than it seems.

Beyond its challenging body mechanics, tai chi requires that you relinquish your reliance on physical energy and instead learn to use your internal energy. To be able to use internal energy you must begin to train your mind as well as your body. The mind is where the power comes from in tai chi. This type of energy is not physical; it is like a gentle internal spiral. You relinquish the physical strength so that later your chi power will increase and flow through your internal channels in a spiral. From that internal spiral comes the true power of the soft way. That's why the power in tai chi uses slow movements. Slow movement increases power.

Also, the slow, continuous, circular movements of form practice allow the healing powers of the flowing chi to help eliminate any blockages, remove imbalances and improve one's overall health. Practicing slowly also cultivates a calmer mind and encourages a more readily attainable meditative mental state which in turn will promote deeper levels of relaxation in the body.

• *The Philosophy of the Soft Way:* Tai chi is a gentle type of physical exercise. As an exercise, it is also related to a specific philosophy. That philosophy tells us that nature's power is soft. To be soft is not necessarily to be weak. There is great power in this softness. This idea, this philosophy comes from nature's way.

The ancient Taoists caught this idea. They tried to discover and learn how to live in this manner. The philosophy of tai chi is something you learn from your own experience, from teaching yourself to be soft. In your daily training, the actions of the tai chi form should be done slowly and your movement should be soft. In moving your body in this slow and deliberate manner over a long period of training, your temperament will gradually become calmer. As a result, you can more readily and easily deal with very tense and suddenly shocking situations. Why? From that daily tai chi form practice, you learn to relax your body and your mind. As a result, this relaxation lesson becomes ingrained in you. After prolonged training, this type of attitude will change your whole life. That's why I think that in the future the beneficial transformative nature of tai chi will become more important in people's lives.

• *Practice the Form from Both Sides:* Traditionally the tai chi form has been taught and practiced from only one side of the body, the right side. This is not surprising since reportedly somewhere between 70% and 90% of all the people in the world are right-handed. Also, the earth turns in only one direction, rivers flow in one direction toward the sea, and clocks only move in one direction. Doubtless, there are many other examples of things that only move in one direction.

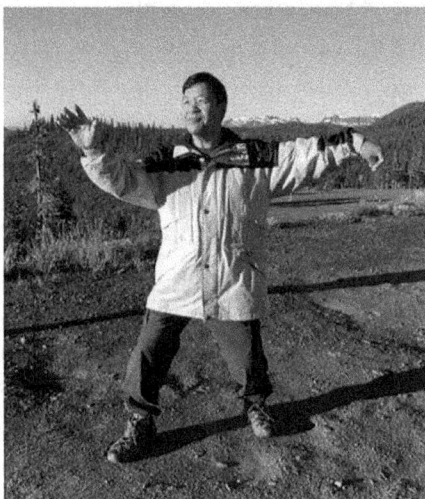

Single Whip, Left Side
Master Wang, Summer Camp Sunrise

However, to only practice tai chi form from the right side is too inflexible. From a martial arts or self-defense perspective you cannot expect an attack from only a right-handed person. You need to be able to defend yourself from all sides. Similarly, in tai chi Push Hands practice it is common to switch which foot is the lead foot when doing fixed-step practice. There are four different combinations possible when doing the "Grasp Sparrow's Tail" sequence with a partner: (1.) Left foot and left arm lead, (2.) Left foot and right arm lead, (3.) Right foot and right arm lead, (4.) Right foot and left arm lead. The actions and responses required are varied in each of the four situations.

But more importantly, if you only practice the form from the right side you contradict the underlying philosophical principle of

Yin/Yang balance. Instead, my students are encouraged to practice their tai chi form on both sides, right and left. To practice in this manner is consistent with the idea of Yin/Yang balance. It will result in improved spatial awareness, better balance, greater coordination, and will make you more accomplished in this art.

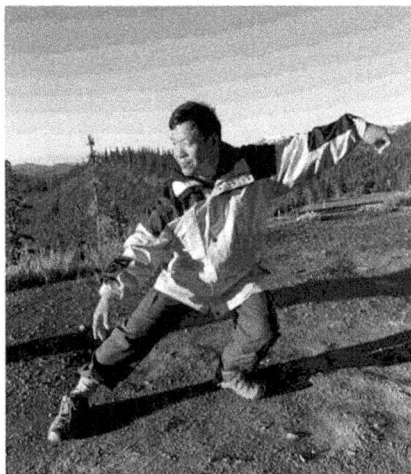

Snake Creeps Down, Left Side
Master Wang, Summer Camp Sunrise

Each of us has one side of the body which is dominant. Thus, we tend to swing a golf club, or hold a baseball bat, or kick a soccer ball, or hold a pencil with one side of the body rather than the other. Except for those few individuals who are truly ambidextrous, when we undertake a familiar action using our non-dominant side we initially perform poorly. We are awkward, unsure, uncoordinated, uncomfortable, and even anxious about our performance. For example, try using your non-dominant hand to write a sentence with a pencil or use a pair of chopsticks.

An added benefit of practicing the form from the left side is the improvement it will give to your brain function. It is well understood that actions performed on one side of the body are controlled by activity that occurs on the opposite side of the brain. There are many exciting new developments in brain function research. Scientists are learning that even as we get older our brains are much more

183

adaptable than previously thought. The brain's plasticity is stimulated by undertaking actions that challenge it to develop new neural connections as a result of being faced with new physical and mental challenges.

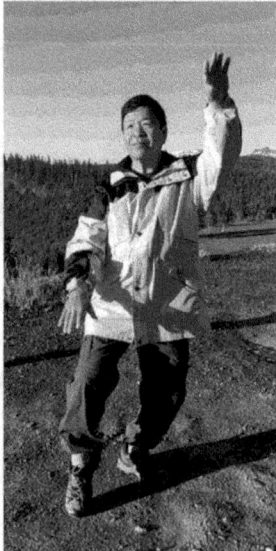

White Crane Spreads Wings, Left Side
Master Wang, Summer Camp Sunrise

On the practical side, over the years I have observed that many people who have practiced tai chi form on just one side have also developed knee pain or suffered knee problems and even injuries that have required surgery. This emphasis of practicing on just the right side places too much weight bearing on one side of the body with no relief. If one of the primary purposes of doing tai chi is to improve your health you need to energize your whole body in the best way possible. By practicing the form on the left side as well as the right side you will obtain better balance of the body, give relief to the potential overuse of the right knee joint and improve the energy of your entire body.

• *Tradition vs. Change:* When I began my practice of tai chi I too was taught in the traditional manner. The forms I learned were all practiced from just one side, the right side. Later I realized that the

184

best athletes in sports such as baseball and basketball can perform their sports from either side. As the practice of tai chi is as much a sport involving physical activity as it is a martial art, it seemed logical that I should begin to practice tai chi from the left side as well as the right. Even though I had this insight, I did not immediately put it into practice since it was not the traditional way of doing things.

In all of the various martial arts, a high degree of respect is paid to the traditions of the art and to preserving the time-tested methods of those who have preceded us. After all, their methods have been proven to be valid time and time again. However, as in other endeavors, there is an inherent tension between preserving the best aspects of the traditional discipline and the need for progress and growth. Too much blind adherence to tradition can result in a stagnant art. One which lacks innovation, development, evolution, or growth. So, eventually, I decided that I should practice on the left side as well as the right.

This has turned out to be the correct decision, both practically and philosophically. Practically speaking it has resulted in my being a more proficient tai chi practitioner because my body and mind are more integrated and able to function equally well on either side. Philosophically speaking, the concept of Yin/Yang balance has been demonstrably preserved as well.

• *Examples from Daily Life:* Let me tell you about three related examples from my own life about our need to adapt and challenge ourselves when faced with new circumstances.

When I moved our family from Taiwan to Vancouver Island none of us had much previous exposure to eating products made from wheat flour. Coming from Asian culture we were used to eating rice and rice products and found them easy to digest. At first, we thought that eating wheat flour products was a crazy notion and felt that they would be hard to digest. Not too long after settling in we began to experiment with this alien Western grain and soon came to enjoy it fully. Fear of change can be difficult to overcome but embracing change can be delicious.

Another example. Growing up in Taiwan I had never been exposed to cheese. There were no Western-style dairy farms and there were no cheesemakers. There was no cheese from buffalo milk or goat's milk in our household either. The only dairy milk I had tasted was powdered milk and I did not much care for it as I found it hard to digest.

When we moved to Vancouver Island, I became fascinated by the many types of cheeses that were available. I had never seen such things nor smelled such interesting aromas. I was, and still am, particularly attracted to those having the strongest odors. Stinky cheeses my children would call them.

However, not having grown up with dairy products as part of my regular diet, I soon discovered that cheese consumption had an unpleasant side effect, diarrhea. My body simply lacked the necessary digestive bacteria or enzymes that were common in my cheese-loving Western students. I tell this somewhat embarrassing story to illustrate my point that our bodies are more adaptable than our minds may realize provided that we are not afraid to make a change. Gradually, I was able to develop a tolerance for cheese products and now it is one of my favorite indulgences.

The final example. As you probably know, the climate of Taiwan is essentially a tropical one. Indeed, the island, which is quite mountainous on the eastern two-thirds, straddles the Tropic of Cancer and the waters surrounding it are correspondingly warm nearly year-round. Imagine my surprise the first time I went swimming in the northern ocean waters which surround Vancouver Island. It was an experience that I did not want to repeat. The water was so very cold!

Even the splendid, inland lakes contained water that felt so chilly to me that I had to practically force myself to wade in. I could not tolerate any of it for more than about ten seconds. I would quickly scramble back to shore and the welcoming warmth of my towel. As my teeth chattered and my toes regained their normal blood flow, I wondered how my students could have enjoyed such a swim. What was normal for them certainly wasn't normal for me.

I decided that since the Comox Valley was my new home, I needed to adapt myself to this new environment. I began taking cold showers. Short ones at first, sometimes very short indeed. However, over about a year I was able to reset my mind's and my body's expectation of what temperature signified cold water. Since then, I can fully enjoy summer swims in the rivers, lakes, and even the oceanside where I live. Again, my point is that the mind and body are more adaptable than you may realize if you don't limit yourself to your preconceived notions and instead allow yourself to make a change.

◆ ◆ ◆

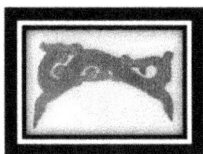

Chapter 11: Three Keys to Tai Chi Form

IT IS MY impression that every generation of tai chi teachers seems to have a different idea about how to optimize the practice of the solo tai chi form. One might say, relax your shoulders. Another might emphasize the development of your root. The next might urge you to loosen the waist and hip joints, the *"kwa"* (kua). Every generation of tai chi instructors mentions a variety of different features or factors concerning the proper execution of the art. For example, among other things, Cheng Man-ch'ing emphasized the importance of maintaining "the beautiful lady's wrist" while doing the form.

I have now accumulated over forty-five years of tai chi practice and experience. At this point, I too have developed my own thoughts about the best and most efficient way to train the body and develop your tai chi form practice. In my judgment, three important characteristics are essential to the correct practice of any tai chi form, regardless of style. Those three necessary elements are: (1.) the position of the head in relation to the trunk, (2.) the operation of the shoulder joint and shoulder girdle, (3.) the management of the *kwa* (kua). or hip joints. Like my Seven Principles, all are equally important.

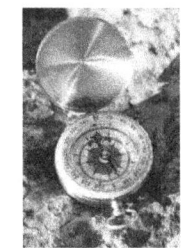

What I have to say may conflict with what others have said in the past. What should you do in the face of conflicting points of view?

If the sources are reliable, you should give them due consideration and seek to give them a fair test of at least a few months' duration or longer in your daily practice. Take a pragmatic approach. See if they are consistent with tai chi's underlying philosophy and see if they work. If they do, then keep them. If they don't, discard them.

Element #1: The Position of the Head

The seven vertebrae of the cervical spine are located in the neck and are the thinnest bones in the spinal column. They enable the head's flexibility, including its rotational, forward/backward, and side bending motions. They also protect the spinal cord and contain openings that allow the arteries that ensure proper blood flow to the brain to pass through.

Most people doing tai chi recognize that the head needs to be held straight and positioned upright, atop the spine. What they may not realize is that according to various authorities, the average, adult human head weighs between eight and eleven or twelve pounds. The brain itself is about three of those pounds. This is a fair amount of weight for the neck to support even when the head is positioned correctly. When the head is held incorrectly, the effective weight which the musculature of the neck has to support increases considerably. Such improper positioning occurs most often when the chin is held in a thrusting forward manner. The greater the deviation from upright the greater the unnecessary load on the head's support system. So, the head should neither tilt forward nor back nor lean to either side. Keeping it balanced properly means that it will be better able to move freely and that the supporting muscles, tendons, and ligaments can more readily relax.

The customary teaching is to move "as if the head is suspended from above". The familiar instructional imagery is that of hanging the body from a string attached to the crown of the head at the Bai-Hui acupuncture point. This is indeed the correct training but the more important concern is how to open the seven joints of the neck (the cervical spine) and keep them loose.

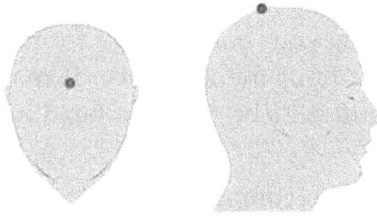

Location of Bai-Hui Point

• *Drop the Chin:* One of the most common corrections that I make to my students is to have them drop their chin just a little. It seems many of them go through their daily lives leading with their chins. This slight forward extension of the chin causes the head to tilt back and an undesirable compression in the cervical vertebrae occurs. In this incorrect position, the muscles, tendons, and ligaments of the neck have to work harder to maintain the balance of the head. By making this rather small and simple correction, there is less tension in the muscles and tissues of the head, neck, and shoulders; and, as a result, the chi is better able to flow up from the spine to the top of the head.

• *Nose and Navel Unaligned*: When doing the form, I tell my students that the torso should turn first and carry the arms. The turning comes from the foot and its root. How does this movement relate to the head and neck? The answer is that rather than keep the head aligned with the stomach (navel) as the body turns, the head should instead remain still at first and then follow slightly after the torso begins to turn. When the torso turns, the head does not immediately go with it.

Let me repeat this instruction which I realize many will find contrary to their established notions and understanding of basic tai chi movement. The common general rule and instruction are to "keep the head aligned with the stomach". By that, it is meant that when the torso turns and changes direction the head should turn at the same time. When following this directive, in a sense, the nose and the navel are kept aligned and move as one. It is my observation that the better practice is to move the torso first and then allow the head to follow a little afterward. While doing every form posture, the head should remain stationary while the torso first starts its rotation beneath it. When doing your entire tai chi form, you should practice this exact way throughout the sequence. It may take considerable practice but the result will be that the head and the neck do not become stiff.

Another false notion common among tai chi players is that the turn of the head should continue and follow the direction of the hand. To my way of thinking, this is also wrong. If the head follows the hand, it is separate from the torso. In tai chi, the softness we cultivate in form practice permits the connection of the internal energy to glide through the body via the rotation of the trunk and the use of the internal spiral. If you use the "head follows the hand" approach the internal energy spiral will be blocked. Remember to tuck the chin slightly. Keep the head straight but the neck joints loose, unrestricted, and moveable. Let the head follow after the torso.

Element #2: Loosen and Open the Shoulder Joints

Tai chi form should be done in a manner that enables the proper opening of the shoulder joints. Relaxation leads to making the shoulder joints loose and open. The shoulder joints support the arms and their movement but these joints can become stiff. When the torso turns the shoulders should be loose. When the torso turns it pulls the shoulders open and loosens them. This in turn enables the connection to the internal spiral action and internal energy. Otherwise, the shoulder joints will be tight, the arms will be stiff, and your form will lack the necessary spiral motion concerning the torso. There are many people who have been doing tai chi form practice for a long time and yet they still have not solved the problem of how to loosen and open the shoulder joints.

Such errors can occur in any posture. For example, many tai chi players have trouble doing the posture "Single Whip" correctly. They are not able to extend the energy upward from the ground and out the fingertips of the bird's beak hand. To test this, a practice partner needs only put light incoming pressure on the bird's beak hand in a straight line toward the torso. When that pressure is slowly increased even a small amount, both people can readily assess whether the body of the person being tested is centered and whether the internal energy is present and connected to the ground at the opposite foot. All too often, the external manifestation of the student's posture may look well-formed but, in reality, it will be what I call "empty". It will lack the key qualitative difference, the felt and evidenced presence of the internal chi energy. This inability can usually be directly traced to the fact that the shoulder and the extended arm of the bird's beak have not been sufficiently loosened and opened. Of course, this is hard to do and requires many hours of the proper type of practice along with gentle testing, accurate feedback, and appropriate corrections.

If you do not open the shoulder joints, the internal chi energy can't travel to and through the bones of the upper and lower arm, wrist, hand, and fingertips. Correct movement while doing the form begins with an upward spiral action that originates from the ground and its energy. The spiraling action that opens upward and outward from the rooted foot is what generates the torso movement, which in turn spirals out the shoulder joint, along the length of the three arm bones, through the wrist joint, and then out and down to the fingertips. This is how you learn to make the internal energy (*nei jin*) which is the demonstration of the internal energy/power at its highest level of achievement.

Element #3: Open Your Hip Joints – The "Kwa"

Mention the *kwa* (kua). to many Western students and you will be met with quizzical looks or even blank stares. They have never heard the word. Of course, to the Chinese, the *kwa* is readily understood as the area of the body surrounding the hip joint and all the related muscles, tendons, and ligaments. The *kwa* includes more than the precise anatomical location which the West identifies as the hip joint. In Western medicine, the hip joint is often described as the ball and socket joint formed by the head of the long thigh bone of the leg (the femur) and the cup-shaped cavity of the hipbone (the acetabulum) where the femur's head connects to the pelvis. To the Chinese, the concept of the *kwa* is somewhat broader and includes the inter-related anatomical structures which surround the joint itself. In simplified Western anatomical terms, the *kwa* would also include the groin area along the crease or hollow of the inguinal fold at the junction between the thigh and the abdomen where the upper leg joins the torso at the lowest part of the abdomen. To the Chinese, the *kwa* involves both function and location. It includes the associated actions involved with the operation of the hip joints in all their normal range of motion as well as the anatomical location. It also can include the simultaneous use of the waist muscles and the leg muscles.

• *Confusing Terms at Times:* It is important to mention that there is a difference between the waist, pelvis (hips), and *kwa*. Sometimes these terms are used interchangeably and that can lead to confusion. In English, the term waist describes the area of the body's trunk which is below the ribcage and above the pelvis. In some translations of Chinese tai chi manuals into English, the word waist has been used to describe what the Chinese consider to be the *kwa*.

In English, the term pelvis denotes the basin-shaped bony structure of the skeleton which connects the upper and lower parts of the body and supports the assortment of internal organs contained in the abdomen. A commonly used synonym for pelvis is hips but that is technically inaccurate. The hips are more properly described as the projecting part of each side of the body formed by the side of the pelvis and the upper part of the femur (the thigh bone) and the flesh covering them. Thus, it is a description of that portion of the hip joint itself which is at the other end of the femoral ball and its socket. It is that area of the body where a tape measurement is taken of "the hips".

• *Moving Together:* When doing the tai chi form, the shoulder joints and the hip joints (or *kwa*) are considered to be interconnected and interdependent. They are often said to operate together. Just like a blocked shoulder joint, if the *kwa* is tight and insufficiently opened you will have the same problem in getting the internal energy to transfer upward from the ground to the torso and then out to the hand and fingertips. Once again, the external look of your form postures can be perfectly correct but if the *kwa* is not opened properly then the energy cannot be transferred through the torso and the spiral cannot go to and from the ground.

Opening the *kwa* is very difficult. In doing your form practice you should "*ti kwa*", or "open the *kwa*". Once the *kwa* is properly opened, you will be able to drop your energy down into the ground and simultaneously transfer energy coming up from the ground through the torso and out the arms, wrists, and fingers. All your tai chi form movements must be done with an awareness of the *kwa's* operation. If you do not move in this mindful way you are not practicing correctly.

In all tai chi form practice, your movements should have a relationship to the pivot of the hip joint. The pivot of the hip joint must remain vertical. The pelvis should remain horizontal. Don't let one side or the other rise up or dip down in a way that disturbs a line where the hips/pelvis remain parallel to the ground.

To maintain the horizontal position of the pelvis you might find it helpful to envision the entire pelvis as a large bowl filled to the brim with water. Your task as you move from posture to posture is to not allow any water to spill from the bowl. There are postures where you are required to bend forward but for most postures, and particularly the transitions between them, the image of the water-filled bowl should help you to maintain the proper position and orientation and to move slowly and smoothly.

In Summary: Three Keys to Tai Chi Form

The following three points are essential for the proper development of your tai chi form practice. Keep the head vertical and let the turn of the torso lead the arms. Loosen and open the shoulder joints. Loosen and open the *kwa*.

Most people who have practiced tai chi for a few years can perform two of these three elements correctly but are not able to work all three together. This is indeed unfortunate because to generate the internal energy (*nei jin*) spiral you must be able to achieve the whole-body coordination of the head, shoulders, and hips. Without attaining this integrated coordination, you cannot properly generate and transmit the spiral energy and there will be no *nei jin*.

The position of the head controls the top level. The shoulder joints control the middle level. The hip joints control the ground level. All three levels must be joined together in combination to produce *nei jin,* the accompanying internal spiral of energy, and the proper build-up of chi. All the movements must be made with the image of the entire body as a "Globe Shape" with the lower dan tien at its center point. (See Chapter 9, "The Seven Principles of Tai Chi", re other references to the "Globe Shape".)

At this point let me assure you that this is not easy to achieve but if you practice with these correct principles in mind it is certainly attainable. You just need to be patient and persistent. In my case, it took me ten years of daily attention, concentration, and effort to coordinate these three levels of the body properly. I believe that Professor Cheng Man-ch'ing and Master Huang Sheng Shyan also struggled in their practice to master this coordination. Do not be discouraged. Instead, be diligent in your practice and the rewards will come.

Remember too that one of the principal reasons to study and practice tai chi is to improve one's health by increasing the store of internal energy. When these three elements are joined together (head, shoulders, and hips) in a coordinated fashion, the chi will generate *nei jin.* Finally, be mindful of my Seven Principles and seek to put them all into play simultaneously as you continue your daily form practice.

The cultivation of proper tai chi form practice is so vitally important. It may take a long time to achieve your goal. Persistence, patience, and principle-based practice are the key to it all. After forty-five years of tai chi experience, both as a practitioner and as a teacher, I still look forward to my regular daily practice which becomes more enjoyable and meaningful day after day.

◆ ◆ ◆

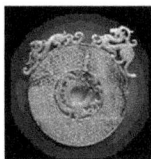

Chapter 12: Transitions & The Chi Trail

IF YOU INCORPORATE the Seven Principles in your tai chi practice you will be able to develop your internal chi energy and you will begin to have the distinct physical sensations associated with the chi moving and circulating throughout your body. As you begin to experience this chi circulation sensation in one or more of the various postures of your tai chi form, you should learn to recognize what I call the "chi trail". This is the next stage in the development of your growth as a practitioner of this internal art.

The concept of the chi trail is the metaphor that I have created and use to explain how to successfully develop, implement, and integrate my Seven Principles into tai chi form practice. I have repeatedly emphasized to my students that it is necessary for them to develop their awareness of the chi trail and to resolve to conduct their daily form practice in such a manner that this trail becomes a well-worn path.

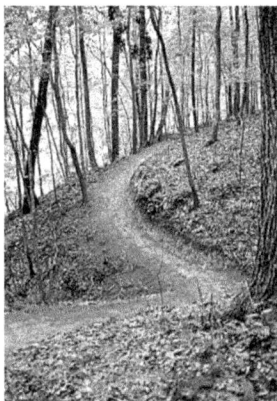

The chi trail is something you develop on the inside of your body. It starts from the bottom of the foot, from your "root", where you connect to the ground's energy. In this context, this ground or earth energy is Yin. Then from the root, you seek to connect this energy through the body to the top of your head at the crown point (bai hui) which connects to the sky/heaven energy.

This sky/heaven energy is Yang. So, you visualize or imagine a link between the root and the crown point through which energy flows. Then you focus your mind in this manner and relax your lower dan tien. The object of this focus is to join together within yourself the energy of the earth and the energy of the heavens. Your relationship to the ground is Yin while your relationship to the heavens is Yang; and, you use the lower dan tien as the place to join them together. When this is successfully done then a third thing emerges as a result of that joinder. That third thing is the chi power available to those who are sufficiently relaxed in the body and sufficiently focused in the mind.

The chi trail is the distinctly detectible internal feeling you get when you can keep the chi moving continuously as you transition your body from one posture to the next. It is a particular qualitative state which gradually develops and is difficult to explain in writing. Generating proper transitions during each of the individual stages of the body's movement from posture to posture is not easy to do. Learning to do it properly is a long process that requires patience and persistence since it cannot be hurried.

Most of the people I have watched practicing the tai chi form over the years are not doing their form practice correctly. They do not pay sufficient attention to maintaining both the "Globe Shape" and "the internal energy trail" or "chi trail". This omission is particularly evident during the stages of their transitional movements from one full posture to the next. They are more concerned with composing the shape of a posture's final position than with anything else. Rather than developing the continuity in the expression of the flow of the internal energy during the transition from one posture to the next, they mistakenly focus their attention on the wrong thing. What occurs during these intervals between postures is extremely important. It is only from maintaining the constant connection of the internal energy to the tai chi trail that internal power is developed and sustained.

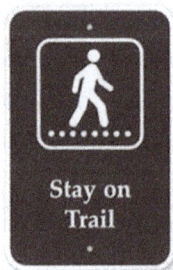

198

When you go trail hiking or trekking, you must walk the entire distance from point "A" to point "B" to point "C" and so on. You do not simply arrive at the trailhead and then expect to be miraculously transported to the first rest area, and then the next, and then the next without any additional effort. Instead, you must do the work and continuously make progress along the chosen route. So too, in doing the form. You have in mind a trail to guide you smoothly from one posture to the next without pause or break. While the body is in motion, the internal chi energy must be fully present and manifested at each point during the transition from one posture to the next; each moment is equally significant to the journey.

There are many people doing tai chi who never reach even the beginning stages of this internal level of development. Certainly, such people can enjoy some benefit from the external physical exercise that they are doing. Making the shapes and repeating the patterned movements they have learned in the form is worthwhile on that level alone. It is a useful physical exercise that improves balance and coordination and provides a host of other effects that are beneficial to health. However, these people are not doing anything more than that. Their form is what I call "empty"; it contains no expression of the internal chi. This is indeed unfortunate.

This trail development in your tai chi form proceeds in three stages. When you begin your training and start to learn and link the individual postures, you must put a considerable amount of conscious thought into the process as you study what each shape looks like, figure out how to construct each shape, and memorize the particular sequence the shapes follow.

Once the appropriate shapes and correct progression of postures have been learned, the next level in your practice then becomes a feeling level. At this stage, you pay more attention to the physical sensations that accompany correct connection throughout the joints of the body and you have less concern with thinking about how to make the shape of a particular posture.

At the third level, you forget completely about thinking about the movement or the associated sensations. At this last stage, the movement occurs spontaneously as a result of the correct alignment and muscle memory you have trained and developed. Your form practice has reprogrammed your central nervous system and fashioned a new set of reflexive responses. The movement becomes embodied in you and becomes your natural way of moving. Right away the proper position and the internal energy are there. At that point, your ability to link the internal energy (*nei jin*) connections of the postures in the form, one to the next, becomes second nature. The chi trail is then a well-worn path.

One example of this embodied movement idea which I often give my students is that of going over to pick up a newspaper off the floor. You don't have to consciously think about how many steps to take, or which hand to reach out, or how to grab it, or how much energy to use to lift it, etc. All those calculations are done automatically and unconsciously. Your mind and hand know what to do. In workshops, I will often place a folding chair in the center of a large circle formed by the group and ask a first-time attendee to walk in and pick up the chair. The puzzled student will easily perform this seemingly pointless task. He or she is always able to go directly to the object, determine its center and balance point, and pick it right up. Anyone doing this doesn't perform a lot of conscious calculations; they simply go do it. This is the same manner in which the chi-filled form is done after a long period of training. It is no longer necessary to think about it. The necessary components have become ingrained and appear spontaneously when the mind directs.

Practicing your form daily can be compared to polishing a piece of jade. Jade in its raw state is just a rather dull piece of stone. It is through the patient work of the artisan that the stone is carved into a harmonious, shining shape. In crafting the stone, the artist does not increase its volume. Instead, after much skillful rubbing and polishing, the stone is worn away until a pleasing shape is revealed. From this patient, gradual erosion, the piece also acquires its luster. This type of discipline is true in all the arts. They all have this one idea in common. The artist needs to practice, practice, practice.

As I've said, by ignoring these three, crucial transitional phases, all of the movements a person makes become merely a repetition of a patterned sequence, one devoid of the internal chi energy. This lack of chi can be readily shown with a simple test. The test involves whether a student can accept the increasing pressure of a slow but steady push applied by their partner to a forearm held in the "Ward-Off" (*Peng*) posture.

When the time comes, those who lack correct alignment and *nei jin* will be unable to accept the gradually increasing pressure of such a slow but steady push.

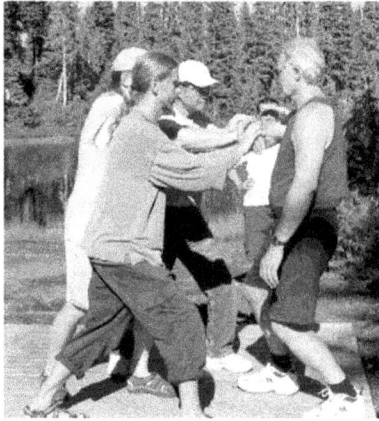

Lawrie Milne "Ward Off" x 3 People

The well-aligned, chi-filled student should be able to accept the pressure of three persons pushing on the "Ward-Off" arm simultaneously. If he or she can do that without physical strain or tension, that is evidence of having attained the proper structural unity inherent in the body's musculoskeletal system. By this I mean the student has been able to achieve the relaxed (*Sung*), interconnected, and properly shaped alignment of the bones, muscles, tendons, ligaments, joints, fascia, and other connective tissues of the body.

Whether you have a traditional, biomechanical view of the body's structure and function or the more recently suggested biotensegrity view of the body's structural reaction to loads and forces, what occurs is not limited by either viewpoint. The student's well-trained stance allows the incoming force to pass through and down into the ground. This result is evidence of the accompanying presence and use of internal energy. Success does not depend on the use of physical strength (*Li*). We work on such things in my classes and at summer camp and many of my students have developed this ability. Here are three other examples.

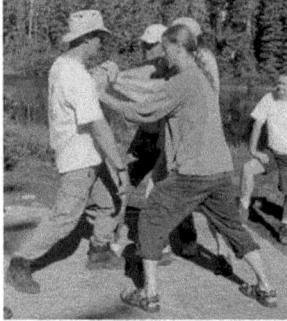
Mike Roach

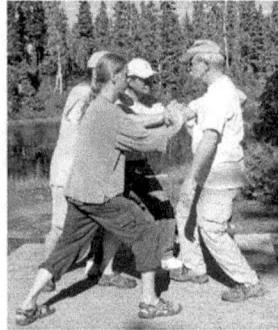
Ted Libby

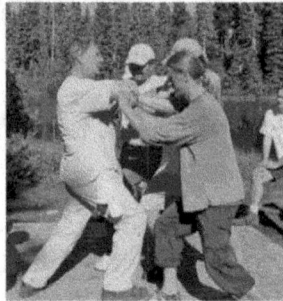
Patrick Deneckere

By doing your form correctly you will increase your internal chi power. This will be readily evident in the "Ward-Off" posture test I've described. But what about in the other postures? Can you hold your shape when placed under a slowly increased amount of pressure? Once you can, there is another level. Can you now release the pressure and project your chi so that your partner is propelled away while your body remains nearly still?

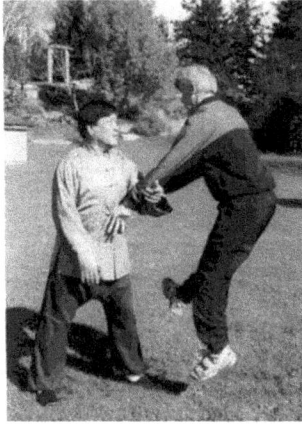

"Ward Off" Demonstration
Master Wang with James Milne

The lowest level in martial arts is that which depends on the use of external physical strength (*Li*), a contest of strength against strength, force against force. The next highest level is that of *Jin* which is not dependent on external physical strength. The *Jin* level relies on relaxed (*Sung*) internal strength and corresponding use of mental imagery in response to the incoming external force.

To be able to hold your tai chi posture while under incoming pressure by use of *Jin* (support without strength or tension) is a correct stage in the development of one's tai chi abilities and an important and significant accomplishment. However, this is only the beginning. It is still a lower level. When you have attained the *Jin* level consistently, the next level becomes the *Chi* level.

But how do you get to that level where internally you have replaced the Jin level with the *Chi* level? You must resolve to spend more time practicing each day. This practice should be done in accord with the Seven Principles and with a mind that is intensely focused on what the principles require as you move through the form or engage with a partner. When your practice is coupled with a keen awareness of whether your actions correspond to those requirements, you will certainly be on the chi trail.

Beyond the *Chi* level, there is the *Yi* or mind/intent level. It may take you ten years of correct work to proceed from level to level. It is a long-term process. Unfortunately, too many people engaged in tai chi are only working at the *Li* level even after many years of practice.

Although my students have often heard these words regarding proper cultivation of the chi trail, in their form practice no one has yet been able to consistently do this completely right throughout an entire round of form. They may get two or three consecutive movements right and connect them correctly; or, they may even string together various distinct segments of the form properly. However, so far, no one has been able to reliably and repeatedly link together and properly connect energetically the entire sequence of postures that the whole form contains. This does not surprise me and it does not discourage them. This degree of dependability is not an easy thing to achieve. It took me many hours of daily practice over a long time to accomplish. Once the Seven Principles are understood it still requires patience and persistence over many years to attain the highest levels of this art.

In my own life, I still perform at least three hours of solo form practice daily. I will usually spend one and one-half hours in the morning and one and one-half hours in the afternoon. Why? Because the transition from one posture to another is so complicated and difficult to master correctly. After forty-five years of practice, I no longer have to think about connecting it. So, in that sense, it is now more spontaneous for me. Nevertheless, I still practice daily in this manner.

As for my students, those who practice regularly and according to the principles are all making noteworthy progress. The other demands of their lives are such that they are unable to devote as many hours to their daily practice as I did and do. Nevertheless, I am pleased to see what they have been able to accomplish and so are they.

Go practice.

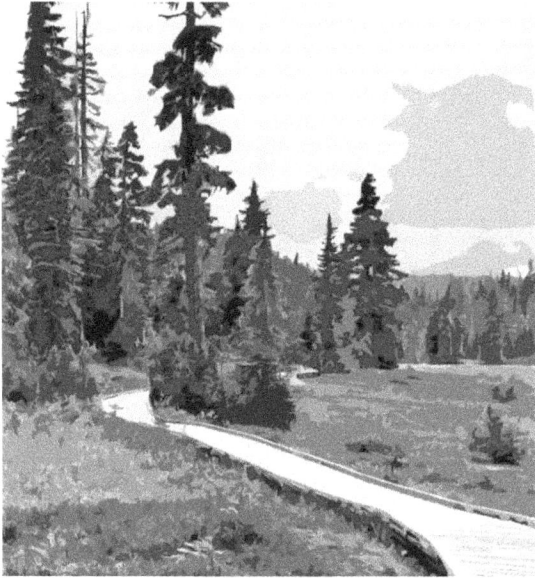

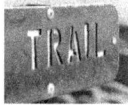

♦ ♦ ♦

尋中道

"Search Center"

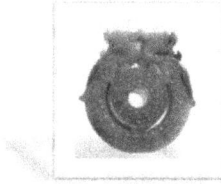

Chapter 13: "Search Center"

A LL NEWCOMERS TO tai chi begin their studies by learning a specific sequence of movements known as the tai chi form. While each style of tai chi has its own distinct form and its own theory and approach concerning how to best perform the art, many postures found in one style are similar if not identical to those found in other styles. What differs from style to style in form practice is the set order of performing the postures, how the body is positioned in particular postures, and which postures are included or subtracted from a given form's routine. Many first-time students gradually lose interest in tai chi and never continue in classes long enough to even learn their particular style's complete set of form postures. For

Search Center a variety of reasons, most students who do learn a particular style's entire routine do not go beyond basic form study to participate in the competitive, partner exercise known as Push Hands (*Tui Shou*).

Traditionally, all tai chi players are told to embody in their form practice the idea that softness overcomes hardness, an idea derived from Taoist philosophy. The imagery of gently flowing water or of a warm summer breeze is often invoked to help convey the desired sense of tranquility, peace, and restorative serenity that is sought.

Students exposed to such ideas and images are better able to practice their tai chi form in the calm, slow, relaxed, and harmonious manner characteristic of the art. However, many of the players who do continue their studies and go on to participate in Push Hands practice quickly abandon their Taoist softness. In doing so, they sacrifice the link between one's tai chi philosophy, individual form practice, and partner practice. This unity of viewpoint is lost and an unwelcome disharmony is introduced as they revert to becoming hard, rigid and unyielding during Push Hands episodes. Invariably, what results is a lack of consistency or compatibility between actions and beliefs, between practice and theory.

• *Push Hands Without Tai Chi Principles:* Push Hands practice is a two-person encounter in which the simple objective is to upset your opponent's balance without losing your own. Upon making contact, the contestants are expected to use a certain set of skills and not engage in a muscle against muscle, force against force struggle. It does not involve punches, strikes, kicks, or throws. Although Push Hands training can be used to provide an introduction to tai chi's martial applications, it is not free-style fighting. To do this correctly, a person should be using the proper body mechanics developed in the form which in turn allow the expression of the internal energy (*nei jin*).

Push Hands lessons usually encourage a participant to relax, to remain mobile, and to lead an opponent into emptiness by not offering resistance to an incoming force. Among other skills, the practice seeks to develop sensitivity, yielding, and neutralizing capabilities. To be successful, you must be able to recognize where in your own body's limbs or joints you are holding tension. The presence of tension will provide your opponent with a direct line to your center of mass and balance. That tension is like a prop holding up a leaning building. When your opponent removes it, your compromised alignment will collapse and gravity will do the rest. You will be tossed out.

Although tai chi is known as a soft style martial art, Push Hands sessions, particularly tournament matches, are highly competitive and can often become overly contentious and even confrontational.

All too often, when faced with a determined attack by a single-minded adversary, tai chi principles are hastily abandoned. The encounter begins with or rapidly escalates to a struggle using muscular, physical force (*Li*). Once a physical struggle develops, the matches quickly deteriorate into a rather inelegant yet aggressive contact sport. This is not correct tai chi.

If you watch a spirited pair in the heat of such an exchange of their supposed soft energy, it may remind you of the children's schoolyard game King of the Hill (a/k/a King of the Mountain or King of the Castle). The object of that game is to stay on top of the high ground while another player attempts to knock you off and take your place. The most widely accepted method of attack is vigorous pushing and shoving but sometimes rougher variations are allowed or do creep in. Since an escalation of violence is likely to occur, many schools ban the game. I believe such pseudo softness needs to be disallowed in Push Hands tournaments as well. But more about banishing certain types of conduct in those tournaments later. (See Chapter 15," Push Hands & The Soft Way".)

Even outside of a competitive tournament match, Push Hands practice itself, regardless of how softly executed, is also inherently competitive. Even if there is nothing more at stake than ego damage, the mindset fostered by this interaction is still one of battle, not relaxation. During tournament competitions, the amount and level of aggressive behavior exchanged by the participants always increase in intensity due to the win/lose nature of such encounters. In saying this, I speak from years of personal tournament experience, not just observation.

I became a Push Hands champion multiple times in Taiwan while still in my twenties. Although at the time I was pleased to have won those tournaments, somewhat to my surprise I found that I was dissatisfied with my accomplishments. Dissatisfied because I knew my victories depended too much on strength and technique and not on the ideal qualities of relaxation and softness expressed in the Tai Chi Classics. I wondered what had happened to the famous tai chi proverb of "four ounces can move a thousand pounds". During those tournaments, the conduct I witnessed, experienced, and even engaged in myself certainly did not embody that philosophy. There was little evidence of that celebrated saying being at all true.

Push Hands practice and competitions reward the development of skill sets that often are contradictory to the underlying philosophy of tai chi. The ability to keep cool, calm, and effective under such competitive pressure is a noteworthy achievement. However, both in the tai chi classroom and in competitions, there is a multitude of incorrect procedures that are encouraged and rewarded. I began to think that there must be a better way to go about things. A way that would be both consistent with tai chi's soft overcomes hard philosophy and still uniquely effective as a means of self-defense.

In 1980, when I first met Grandmaster Huang, Sheng Shyan of Malaysia, I recognized that I had finally come across someone who possessed the true skills associated with the soft style of martial arts. I studied with Master Huang whenever he visited Taiwan. Taking inspiration from him, I was later able to discover for myself the secrets of attaining this soft power. Wanting to emphasize softness rather than strength and the use of internal chi energy rather than physical force, I named my new method "Search Center". When engaged in "Search Center" practice I use internal chi energy rather than external muscular force to move my partner. Those who are well trained in "Search Center" are capable of using their internal chi energy in the same manner as I do.

- *A Wuwei Alternative to Push Hands:* Push Hands is an agreement exercise in the sense that there are rules as to what type of actions can be taken. As I've mentioned, there are no punches, no strikes, no kicks, no throws, no foot sweeps, etc. However, under the current rules, the main shortcomings of Push Hands are that it encourages confrontation, rewards aggression, and lacks cooperation.

"Search Center", on the other hand, is a principles-based, training method developed to take the physical struggle and the use of strength out of Push Hands interactions. "Search Center" reintegrates partner practice with both individual form practice and

212

tai chi theory/philosophy. It restores the unity of this trio of tai chi's essential elements by encouraging consistent thought and behavior in all three aspects of one's tai chi practice.

The philosophical basis for tai chi follows the teachings of Lao Tse, and particularly the concept of Wuwei. The term Wuwei can have different meanings depending on the context. On a political scale, it is often associated with how to construct the ideal form of government. On a personal level, Wuwei is often associated with the idea of non-action or passivity but that is an incorrect understanding. Although it does seek to be non-oppositional in response to existing circumstances, Wuwei also emphasizes the Taoist outlook that in any situation one should act naturally and appropriately, at the right time and manner. In the practice of tai chi, the implication would be that the actions taken would not involve a struggle but would instead simply be natural, harmonious, and unforced.

My "Search Center" idea seeks to incorporate this particular outlook and philosophical interpretation of the principle of Wuwei. By practicing tai chi in accord with my Seven Principles you will attain the consequential awareness, confidence, and tranquility that results from the persistent practice of any learned skill. To have Wuwei in this context is then to be able to act spontaneously and without a preconceived purpose. That is, as a result of your training, you are capable of responding competently and appropriately as the situation warrants but do so without a preplanned, specific, inflexible goal in mind.

My "Search Center" method of practice is the expression of Wuwei not Yo Wei in partner work. In Yo Wei you have a preplanned purpose. In "Search Center", you don't act with a purpose in mind. By this, I mean that your goal is not to defeat your partner. Your goal is to understand his or her energy and how your energy is reacting and responding in the face of it. You seek to understand your partner's energy and whether you have the skills to cope with it. Ultimately, you seek to interact with his or her energy in such a manner that your partner defeats himself or herself due to their ambitious actions.

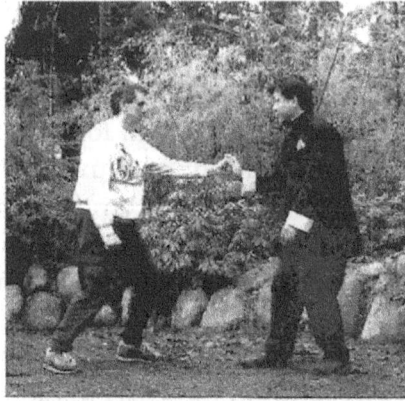

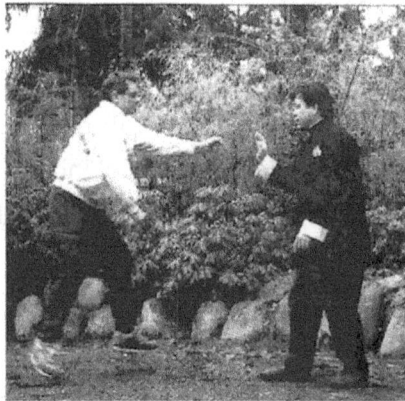

Peter Uhlmann & Master Wang

In "Search Center", when you first make physical contact with someone, that initial sensation of touch should immediately convey what is truly happening between you. You should understand the state of your own body's response to that touch and recognize your problematic reactions. You need to realize whether you are stiff, tight, or have not dropped your weight into the ground to establish a good root. Whether your sensitivity to the situation is sharp or dull should be immediately apparent to you but, hopefully, not so readily apparent to your partner. From all this information, you should try to improve yourself by reading and responding to the message sent by the other person.

The "Search Center" training method rejects the idea of competitive struggle. Instead, partner practice becomes more a cooperative/collaborative exercise in learning, understanding, and improving your own and your partner's abilities. It uses the practice of the traditional tai chi form postures primarily as a means to cultivate the required softness and as a way to connect to and embody Lao Tse's philosophy. In this manner, it leads to a soft martial arts solution. This approach also builds up a more spiritual and harmonious path for both participants. A path such as this is a more appropriate one for the 21st century. I believe that we in the tai chi community should consider that it is now time to make such a change.

This book will introduce you to these ideas and this method of training. I hope that you will be encouraged to explore these ideas and experiment with these methods in your tai chi practice. The time spent in this method of training will certainly produce health benefits, rejuvenate the body and spirit, and promote longevity. Faithful practice will also better enable people to maintain their independence in old age. Also, for those interested in the self-defense aspects of tai chi, "Search Center" can provide an effective response to aggression and do so in a manner that is consistent with the soft way.

• *Repositioning the Practice Partners:* In the usual manner of fixed-step Push Hands, the players both assume an Archer's Stance and then line up with their front feet placed toe to heel. In "Search Center", both players also take an Archer's Stance but the players' front feet line up toe to toe on either side of an imaginary line drawn on the ground between them. Their toes must never cross that line.

From this starting position, the "Search Center" players are standing farther apart. This makes it much more difficult for them to physically manhandle each other without compromising their own balance. This positioning is intentionally designed to frustrate Push Hands players who are using brute, physical strength to throw out their partners.

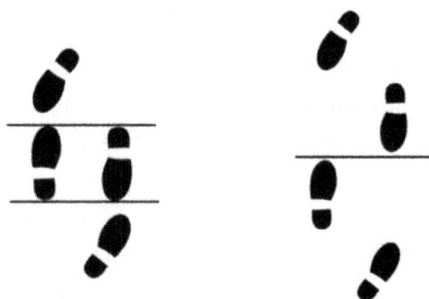

Push Hands Stance   "Search Center" Stance

Each player adopts an Archer's Stance with centerlines facing so the navels point directly at each other. To begin constructing a proper Archer's Stance, a person stands with toes pointing forward, both feet parallel, and positioned shoulder-width apart. Then, while maintaining the shoulder width throughout, he or she takes a step forward with one foot which continues to be pointed straight ahead. The other foot (which is now the rear foot) remains in its original position but is pivoted on its heel until the toes are turned and pointed out at a forty-five (45°) degree angle. The hips and trunk are then squared up so that the navel and head are pointing in the same forward direction as the front foot. My method allows and encourages the weight to be kept evenly divided on both feet, 50/50 while standing in this position. As explained elsewhere, this weight distribution does not result in a forbidden, double-weighted situation which all styles of tai chi caution against.

Since I originally introduced this change in the stance distance between the partners, "Search Center" practice has evolved in ways I never expected. It has become more of a collaborative exercise than Push Hands tends to be. That does not mean that "Search Center" is only done cooperatively. It can also be done less cooperatively and more competitively. But I hesitate to even use the word competitive to describe what occurs because you, as the reader, will probably have a mental image that involves confrontation, struggle, and fighting, etc. That is not what occurs.

There are various levels to this "Search Center" type of partner work and my more advanced students are more adept at understanding what is required under various conditions, including encounters with more forceful and competitive partners. Because learning not to use physical force is so difficult, at the outset the best way to learn the use of internal energy is through interactive cooperation rather than confrontation. This is a valuable lesson in many of life's other contexts as well. There will be plenty of time later to test your soft, internal energy skills with an antagonistic, non-collaborative partner. There is no shortage of them.

For too many years now, the widespread practice has been to conduct the performance of the form according to tai chi principles only to see adherence to those principles ignored and abandoned in Push Hands. Abandoned because they are considered impractical. People seem to believe that for Push Hands it is necessary to build a strong root and fight back. As a result of adopting such a mistaken approach, the philosophical principles of tai chi and the activities taking place during Push Hands have become unrelated. This is a grave error.

In "Search Center", we do not proceed in that manner. We instead insist upon and continue to train in the use of the soft way. "Search Center" is the correct extension of the soft philosophy into soft action. It enables the effective outward expression of a person's accumulated internal energy. The internal energy obtained as a result of their principles-based form practice. Using the soft way, one develops the ability to feel, know, and respond harmoniously to adversity and aggression. This is a different strategy from that found in hard-style martial arts with their emphasis on the use of aggressive fighting to defend oneself. The soft manner in which "Search Center" practice develops teaches one how to yield and occupy one's partner's space in a way that efficiently and effectively neutralizes his or her efforts. Ultimately, all you need to know and master is how to yield to strength and how to simultaneously occupy and thus control the partner's center. That's all you need to do. If you can do this, partners will soon find that they are unable to win this game.

With perhaps just five months of training, you can understand the principles of "Search Center" practice and how it should work.

However, it is likely to take you at least five years or more to embody those principles and begin to make them work effectively. The acquisition of these skills is not instantaneous. It takes considerable time and, particularly at the outset, the right kind of practice with a knowledgeable, collaborative partner.

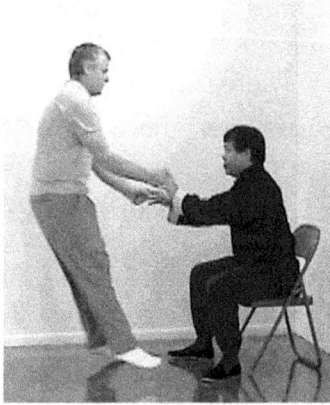

Seated "Search Center", Master Wang

• *Playing the "Search Center" Way:* In "Search Center" there are no fancy hand movements. There is no extended partner interplay like that found in the two-person, four-posture, "Grasp Sparrow's Tail" exercise sequence commonly used in the Cheng Man-ch'ing schools and some other schools as well. There is no set pattern to "Search Center" either. There is only sensation and what results from that sense of awareness. When doing "Search Center" there is no concern about following the traditional "eight directions" or "eight gates" that we practice in the tai chi form and no plans to make use of their corresponding martial arts applications. The eight directions are: (1.) Ward Off (*Peng*), (2.) Rollback (*Lu*), (3.) Press (*Ji*), (4.) Push (*An*), (5.) Pull-Down (*Tsai*), (6.) Split (*Lieh*), (7.) Elbow or elbow strike (*Chou*), and (8.) Lean Forward or shoulder strike, (*Kao*). Similarly, the five steps common to the various tai chi styles are not featured. The five steps are: (1.) forward movement, (2.) backward movement, (3.) move or look to the left, (4.) move or look to the right, and (5.) central equilibrium. While these thirteen features of tai chi are directly related to aspects of Taoist philosophy so is the "Search Center" training.

There is no attempt to turn "Search Center" partner work into an applied martial art. We only practice from sensation and, at first, we tell each other what is right or wrong about the interaction. When you are first learning to conduct a search, your partner will listen and tell you how effective you are in locating/identifying his or her center point. Initially you just make light contact, hand to hand, and try to feel whether you've established a connection to your partner's center, and vice versa.

In "Search Center", you try to accurately find your partner's center point. This is very different from a Push Hands encounter. In this way of practice, you seek to join with your partner rather than push him or her. If you find the partner's "hard" part, you will have found the center. If you can control that center point, he or she will be out of balance. At the higher level of achievement, instead of finding hardness, you will be able to find an empty spot. That empty spot is the true center. After lots of practice, you will be able to realize quite readily when and where this occurs. At the first touch, you will be able to find and control their center point.

There are four factors or components involved in each "Search Center" interaction: (1.) The degree of relaxation you can manifest and maintain upon making contact with your partner; (2.) The extent of your ability to yield to an incoming force or incoming search and your ability to use and develop the internal spiral in doing so; (3.) The level of your sensation and sensitivity to your own and your partner's energy and the ability to search another's center without revealing your own; (4.) The extent of your ability to use the mind/intent (*Yi*) to project your internal chi power effectively.

In your training practice, you will learn to conduct a search and to defend against such a search. In mounting your defense, the key skills are to listen, yield, and relax. This is how you should train. Let the partner search you and see if you can accept and thereby neutralize their search. At the same time, you can study your listening ability, the depth of your root, the reciprocal sensation between you and the other person, your sense of balance and that of your partner, and your mutual extension of chi energy. It is completely absorbing to train in this manner and very enjoyable as well.

You also get more health benefits from "Search Center" practice than from Push Hands practice. Push Hands involves a contest to see who can yield quickly and then push back. As a result, people develop tension and a hyper-alert fight or flight consciousness which makes it difficult to relax and remain calm. The body and the mind both become reactive, nervous, and tense. Such an outcome is the opposite of the state of relaxation which is encouraged and cultivated during solo tai chi form practice.

• *How "Search Center" Training Begins:* Whether you are engaged in form practice or partner work, your Center must initiate all movement. The lower dan tien is both the storehouse of your chi and the location of your Center. Therefore, the very first step in any "Search Center" interaction is to be in your Center. Being in touch with your Center is a subtle but actual physical sensation that requires training to recognize. You cannot hope to use your internal energy effectively against someone else if you are not moving from your Center. If you cannot reliably find the storehouse, how can you ever hope to use the contents?

The ability to be in touch with your Center is learned through the practice of the tai chi form diligently and attentively over and over again. This requires extensive, carefully crafted repetition to produce a very accurate and precise execution of the postures and the transitions between them. We practice with precision to attain the ability to consistently recognize and reliably find our Centers. In turn, such practice will increase our confidence that we are capable of doing what is required.

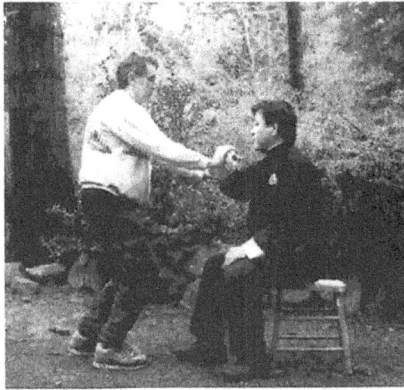

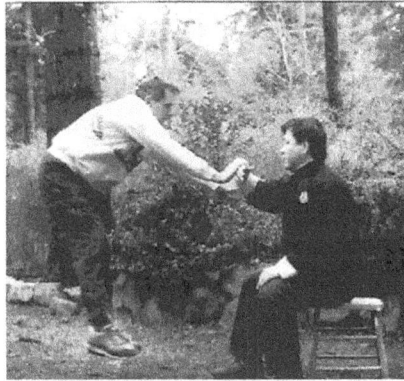

Peter Uhlmann & Master Wang

We also need to develop listening energy (*ting jin*) to know the awkward parts of our bodies and those of our partner's bodies. Our bodies have a certain innate internal harmony (feng shui) which is in accord with nature's way. If the various parts of the body are out-of-place during form practice, the body's natural feng shui can be disrupted and the performance can feel awkward. For example, if the spacing of the footwork is incorrect when changing directions or when making a transition between postures our maintenance of the Center will be compromised. We practice the form repeatedly to recognize the correct placement of the feet and to recognize the incorrect placement. As we move through the tai chi form, we seek to find harmony with nature in our movements and our lives.

You too can find this correct understanding for yourself just as I did. In my case, I did it in part by studying nature, sports, martial arts, Taoist philosophy, and traditional Chinese medicine. Experience is the teacher. Some people are naturally more talented at doing this than others and so catch this idea sooner. But, in the long run, this does not matter as most everyone can achieve the correct result. It just means that others may have to work longer and harder.

• *Finding Your Center:* Many players who have been practicing tai chi form and Push Hands for years have no well-developed sense of the internal feeling which is properly associated with their Center. In most cases, this is because they have never practiced their tai chi form in the correct manner which would put them in their Center. Even those who may have attained a Center often simply do not recognize it, let alone, understand its importance. They don't catch the feeling of the Center.

What does it mean then to be in your Center? How will you know? As mentioned earlier, the related sensations are very subtle and hard to recognize at first. As you begin to learn this approach to partner practice, the surest way of knowing whether you are moving from your center point is by having a cooperative partner confirm it for you. Acting from the Center is what makes the energetic connection to another person possible. If your partner confirms that you have indeed made an energetic connection with them then you necessarily must be acting from your Center. When this connection is confirmed, you should carefully study the positioning and sensations occurring in your own body; and, then seek to reproduce similar feelings during the next attempt to connect with your partner. Similarly, when doing your solo form practice you should systematically assess whether the postures and the transitions produce that same internal state. After some time and practice, this ability to know when you are acting from your Center will become automatic in your form and your partner work. You will know when you have successfully connected.

When first learning "Search Center" my students often comment that it is much easier for them to sense an effective connection and search when they act as the recipients rather than being the sender/searchers. For some reason, when acting as sender/searcher, it is more difficult for them to recognize when they have correctly performed an effective search and made a successful connection. A comment often heard from a beginner who has just moved their partner as a result of having conducted a successful "search" is: "But I didn't do anything!"

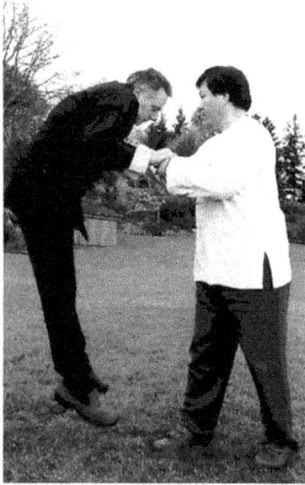

Peter Uhlmann & Master Wang

A sender/searcher's role is the more active one. The sender/searcher must organize his or her mind (*Yi*/intention) and body (attentive action) to obtain a center-based connection to their partner. He or she must also recognize that the connection has occurred. Moreover, the connection and the recognition of it must be established at the moment of the first touch. It should occur when the recipient initiates the initial contact with the sender/searcher. Thus, being a sender/searcher is more difficult at first. The fact that there is such an elusive and refined degree of sensitivity required is why the attainment of this level of awareness by each "Search Center" partner, is more readily trained through cooperative/collaborative rather than uncooperative/competitive practice. This is particularly true for the "sender/searcher".

• *Connecting to Your Partner:* Having first developed the sensation of your Center, the next step in this interaction is to connect your Center to that of your partner. To do so you must first be in your Center. Then you must be sensitive and able to feel your partner's Center. This does not mean that you have to actually lay hands on their lower dan tien or even touch the midline of their body. It means that from the moment of the initial point of contact you are immediately able to sense and feel the direction of an imaginary straight line leading directly from that point of contact to their Center, the location of their exact point of balance. When doing "Search Center", you use your hand to "mark" that point of your partner's centerline, and then you do not move your hand in space at all. Instead, you focus your mind and extend your chi energy thru that hand on the imaginary straight line you feel to their Center.

In "Search Center" practice, you consciously make use of correctly composed tai chi form postures and give up the physical strength which is so often manifested in their use during regular Push Hands practice. What you give up in relinquishing physical force you will immediately gain in sensitivity and listening energy, tai chi's *ting jin*. To develop *ting jin,* you must resolve to relax the body *(Sung)* and focus the mind (*Yi*). Doing so is the entry point for learning this skill. Without relaxation or focus it is impossible to implement *ting jin* at the level which "Search Center" requires. Both characteristics must be present simultaneously. You are now playing a different game from the one played in most Push Hands situations. One of the main goals of "Search Center" practice is to regain the unity between the philosophy of tai chi and the embodiment of that philosophy in the tai chi form. The mind, body, and philosophy must be united harmoniously.

Since for beginners, this type of partner work training is cooperative at first, both players are encouraged not to "hide" their Centers from their partners. Keeping your Center available for your partner to locate will speed up the learning process and is beneficial to both players. Proceeding in this manner will permit the sender/searcher to locate what needs to be found and will at the same time allow the recipient to recognize when their Center has been located and compromised.

Although one person will act as the sender/searcher and the other will act as the receiver during the initial training phase, in the final analysis, it does not matter who originates that first physical touch. Once making physical contact, no matter how light the touch, you must immediately know where that vulnerable point of your partner's balance is located. As well as the feedback from physical touch, a connection also involves concentration and use of the mind/intent (*Yi*). This is much easier to write about and explain conceptually than it is to do.

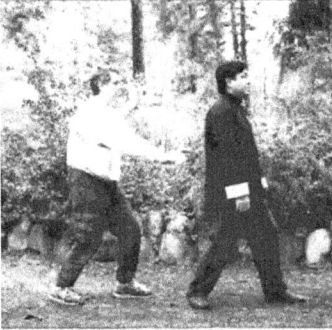

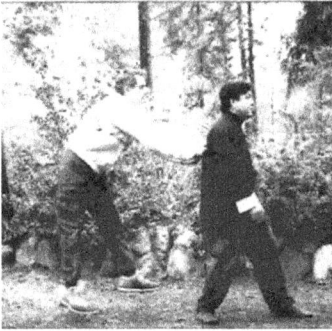

Since the initial understanding of what's involved is so subtle and perhaps counter-intuitive or counter-instinctual, it would be more beneficial if persons who are new to "Search Center" could first be partnered with more experienced

Peter Uhlmann & Master Wang

players who are familiar with its nuances. Two novices attempting this type of work together will not as readily understand what is being asked and may soon become frustrated.

Years of experience in teaching this method to my students and in watching them struggle to learn it has exposed perhaps the most common problem for beginners. A person new to searching is most often completely unable to reliably find their partner's Center even when it is wholeheartedly offered. Having a more experienced recipient verbally confirm whether or not a proper connection has been made is essential to the "Search Center" learning process.

Receiving encouragement and accurate feedback is an important part of successful training.

Coincidentally, because the partners are engaged in the mutual goal of making and recognizing when a connection has occurred the sense of camaraderie and friendship between them also tends to grow. On the other hand, if the recipient's Center is actively concealed the beginner may never understand the task and miss the point of the exercise entirely. So, the more satisfactory training method is to not hide the Center until a player has become reasonably proficient at searching. Only then should the stakes be increased by the recipient's sinking, concealing, or withdrawing their Center so it becomes harder to find. Skilled players can hide their Centers entirely and consequently can draw their partners into emptiness and a resultant loss of balance.

"No Center, No Balance.
No Balance, No Power."

Interestingly, if the connection is done correctly no amount of wiggling or other types of evasive maneuvering by your partner will be able to dislodge you from their balance point. Once captured by you, it is your goal to retain that center point connection but without struggling to do so. It is not done with physical strength. If your opponent moves your limbs or torso in some physical way to shake you off you have a choice. You can let it happen or you can neutralize their energy and respond with your internal chi to disrupt their balance, compromise their root, and thus cause them to "lose". Lose what? The equilibrium of their center point.

Gravity is constantly exerting a downward pull on our bodies. When centered the body has a largely unconscious capacity to maintain balance in response to that gravitational force. When we conduct a search successfully gravity becomes our ally as we disrupt our partner's Center. Without a center point, there is not nor can there be any balance. What necessarily follows is a collapse and a fall until the body attains a new, stable relationship with gravity. As I frequently tell my students, "No center, no balance. No balance, no power."

• *The First Priority is Ting Jin:* Having now found your partner's Center, the next thing you must do is recognize, absorb, and neutralize any incoming physical force (*Li*) directed towards you. You must not respond to their use of force with force. Your hands are used primarily as antennae to sense another person's energy, not as instruments to push. Complete neutralization must occur before you emit your chi outwards. This capacity develops in connection with your attainment of a more refined *ting jin* (listening energy).

As you develop your *Ting Jin* abilities you will go through several different stages, each more sensitive than its predecessor. The stages, from stiff and hard to supple and soft can be characterized or described as follows: (1.) wood, (2.) bamboo, (3.) paper, (4.) cotton, (5.) wool, (6.) silk, (7.) water, and (8.) air. When encountering a hard force, each of these stages denotes a greater ability to yield and offer less and less resistance while absorbing and thus neutralizing that force. Soft overcomes hard.

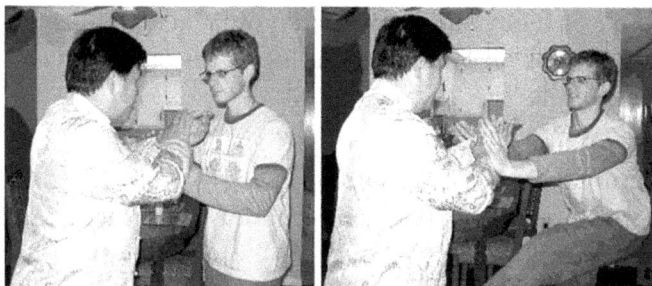

"Search Center" in Press (Ji) Posture
Master Wang & Chris Bryhan

The person whose Center you have connected to does not feel any pushing or pain upon contact. When the internal energy is transmitted it feels to them more like being moved backward by a large, gentle wave of wind or water. Gentle but powerful and still quite impossible to resist. Perhaps the most interesting aspect of this phenomenon is that while they are being uprooted, the first part of the body to move is usually the center area not the point of contact.

227

Once a recipient's center point is successfully compromised, they tend to collapse or bend at the waist. It can look like he or she has just received a strong punch to the lower belly or as if they have been yanked backward by a sharp pull from behind.

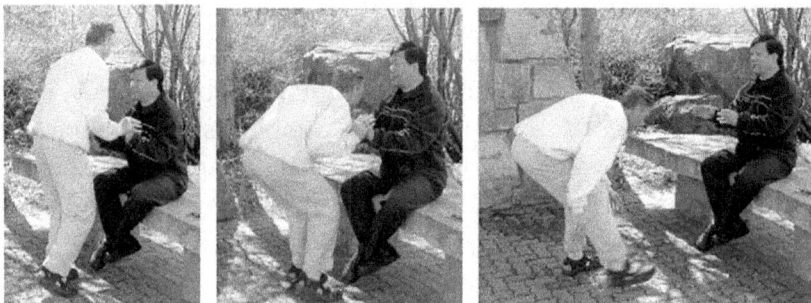

Master Wang & Paul Seronko. Master Wang's feet are off the ground.

• *The Levels of "Search Center" Play*: The practice of "Search Center" has different levels of accomplishment within it. These are the various stages you will encounter in your partner work. It is unlikely that you can proceed to a higher level without going through all of them one by one. As you practice more you begin to attain a deeper level of understanding of the subtle layers of internal energy cultivation.

Level #1 The "Li" Detection Level via "Ting Jin": The initial level is the familiar *Ting Jin* (listening energy) level. This refers to the correct interpretation of the information obtained from the initial sensation of any hand-to-hand touch between two players. You can eventually learn to listen with your whole body. Most people who have engaged in Push Hands practice or any other partner work have at least some passing familiarity with the term *Ting Jin*.

The "Search Center" idea is that when you touch the opponent with the back of your hand you are to use that contact point to establish a relationship with your partner and simply make a horizontal circling motion by rotating the body using your lower dan tien (hips/pelvis). Try to use the sensation at the point of contact to find the partner's Center. As you circle, act without any desire or purpose to push or grab the partner. From the moment of initial contact, you listen to your partner's *Li* (muscular or physical strength). You should also try to yield, avoid, and not resist his or her *Li*. The more you practice the more your level of accomplishment improves and the more successful you will become at neutralizing *Li*. "Search Center" at the *Ting Jin* level has to start at the outer surface, at the level of muscles, strength, and physical force. This is where you will always find and can feel your partner's *Li*.

Level #2 The "Jin" Level: You next learn to listen to your own and your partner's "*Jin*" level. This is a high level of inside strength; not outside strength. At the *Jin* level, you feel his or her tendon. You find your partner's Center and try to avoid revealing your own Center. You do this by being softer than your partner. You don't want people to hear/sense your *Jin* and Center. When working at this level it is difficult to hide your own Center and *Jin*. Later you become very gentle and the touch's contact point with your partner becomes very light.

Level #3 The "Chi" Level: At this level, you can find your partner's Center even before he or she moves. At the same time, you won't want to expose your own direction of movement, Center, and *Jin*. You have now become very gentle and, at the same time, your touch is very light.

At the Chi level, you sense whether your partner has movement. You also sense the related motivation or intent. You can sense when your partner is about to move before his or her movement begins. You are already a step ahead. This takes lots of practice. Your sensation becomes very sharp. This is how you get the hang of the "right timing" aspect of your response to your partner's efforts. At the Chi level, you are almost feeling the inside of your partner's bones.

Level #4 The "Yi" Level: At the *Yi* level, hand-to-hand contact is not necessary. Without it, you can nevertheless "feel" a person's intention and your Center can already start to yield. You feel inside your partner's mind. By doing "Search Center", you can find the "currents" of impending movement before the actual movement occurs. You can break the line between Shen and Chi.

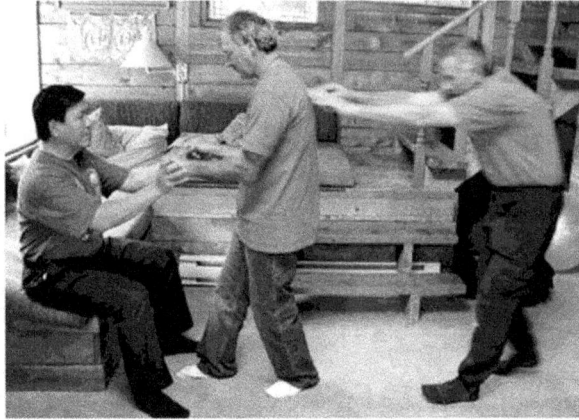

"Search Center" Through Two People
Master Wang, Bill McKee & Peter Uhlmann

• *"Search Center" Requires Mental Focus:* To make progress in your tai chi practice you cannot let your mind become rigid and locked into preconceived notions and ideas about what tai chi practice is or is not. You will never be able to open the gate leading to the development of internal power without first having the right key. The key to this internal development is the proper use of the mind in coordination with the body. (See Chapter 8, "Development of Internal Chi").

During "Search Center" training, people can rather quickly understand the idea of what is required but are simply unable to put it into practice. The principal reason for this gap between the intellectual understanding of what needs to occur and the actual implementation of proper action is the lack of sufficient internal relaxation *(Sung)* to permit the unrestricted flow of chi. To achieve success in "Search Center" you first need to achieve a state of overall relaxation in the body *(Sung)* but also in the mind. For *Sung* to develop properly, you must instruct the mind to work on three essential tasks: (1.) the need to give up fear, (2.) the need to give up the desire to win, (3.) the need to persist and grow in one's practice. It will be impossible to relax sufficiently without training the mind in these fundamentals; and, without the prerequisite relaxation, it will be impossible to project chi energy.

To put the mind in its proper state you must be able to control your fear and apprehension when standing face to face with your partner during "Search Center" or Push Hands practice. You can't allow yourself to be anxious or concerned about whether that person is bigger, stronger, faster, or more experienced than you are. When pushed, the only thing that you should concern yourself with is your ability to use the soft way of interaction. Just practice your tai chi by following the Seven Principles. In this way, your tension and anxiety will be dissolved and your composure, confidence, and self-reliance will be improved.

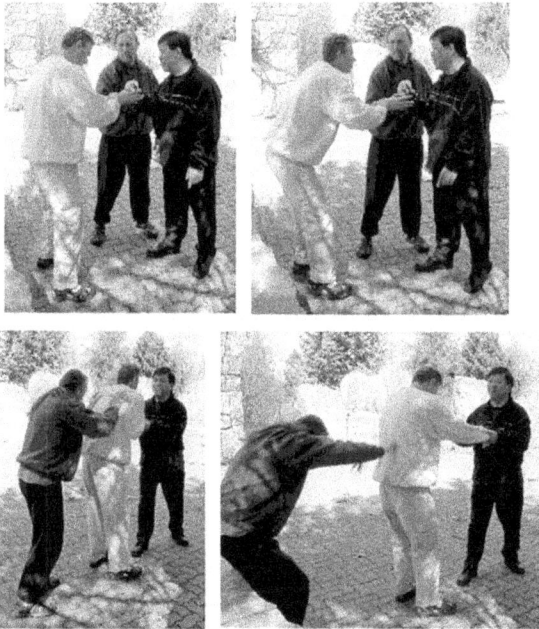

"Search Center" Through Two People
Master Wang, Paul Seronko & Greg Harley

To keep your mind in a proper state you must also realize the necessity of keeping your ego in check. When engaged in a "Search Center" or Push Hands session you should never think that you are better than your opponent or that you will be the winner. After all, what is it that you have won exactly? Instead, you should focus on yielding to the situation at hand. Even as your successes in "Search Center" or Push Hands encounters improve (perhaps you have even won in various tournament competitions), you must remain humble and not take undue pride in your accomplishments. Don't use your powers against people or fight with people. Let your ego go. Let any conceit and sense of self-importance go. Remind yourself that the study of tai chi can be a bountiful, life-long undertaking that will also provide numerous health benefits as well as many fine friendships with other like-minded people.

Everyone knows that becoming proficient in any skilled undertaking requires dedication and hard work. This is what the phrase "kung fu" means. Such kung fu is certainly required to achieve a high level in tai chi. Therefore, to keep your mind in a proper state you must also realize that regardless of how successful you become in "Search Center" or Push Hands practice there is always more to learn and more to study. One of the most appealing aspects of tai chi practice is that it is truly open-ended. There is no set limit to how much progress can be made. There is always the challenge of getting even softer and yielding more. After over forty-five years of practice, I am still constantly learning, still engaged in kung fu.

"Yong Yi, Bu Yong Li."

• *An Exercise for "Search Center" Beginners:* Try practicing in this simple manner at first. Select a like-minded partner, one with considerable experience if available, and begin a "One-Hand Circling" exercise. Use only the back of the hands as the point of contact between you. As there are fewer nerve endings and touch receptors there than in your fingertips this is a greater challenge to your listening abilities. Just maintain that hand-to-hand contact as lightly as possible and see if you can find your partner's Center. See if you can understand what that means. Relax (be *Sung*) and listen to your partner with an attentive sensation of touch, your *ting jin*; and, listen as well to the verbal feedback you receive concerning whether you are on your partner's Center or not. The beauty of this simple exercise is that when properly performed it is so clear in the outcome. There are only two possible results. Either you have your partner's

Center or you don't. What could be simpler? What could be more challenging? (See Appendix "A", "One Hand Circling".)

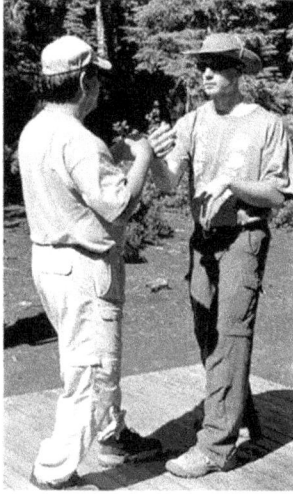

"One Hand Circling"
Master Wang & Chris Bryhan

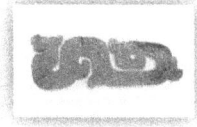

Chapter 14: "No-Touch" Work

A S I BEGIN this discussion of "No-Touch" it is perhaps good to recall that in all types of martial arts there is an inherent tension between respecting and following the teaching methods and lessons of your master and the need for innovation and progress in

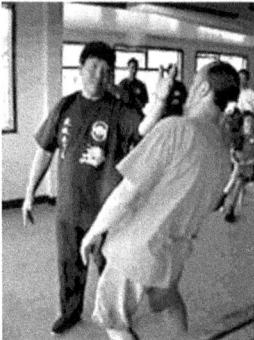

Master Wang & Greg Harley

the art. The traditional method of teaching and learning martial arts puts a great emphasis on the need to respect the lessons and tradition handed down from your teacher. This respect is an important aspect of martial arts culture and tradition but it can result in the development of ideas that become frozen in time. So, while strict adherence and respect for traditional teachings is one way to go, I believe that developing and advocating for a change of methods while still maintaining and adhering to the foundational principles is another way to go. When adopting this attitude there is no less respect but there is now room for growth, innovation, and progress.

• *Mind Closed or Mind Open:* For example, I have posted several videos on YouTube in which I demonstrate the "No-Touch" or "Without Touch" use of soft chi power to toss a person away. My students and those who have attended my workshops or summer camps will readily attest that this power and ability are real. Yet the comments these videos receive are mostly negative. People who have never met me or who never experienced this soft power from other high-level tai chi players say that the videos are fake, or magic, or hypnosis, or only work on my students. They are unable to believe that "without touch" is possible.

They are certainly entitled to their opinions. But this is also a good example of people who are trapped in their preconceived notions and ideas about chi power. They become frozen in their beliefs and unable to acknowledge even the prospect that such things may be possible. People whose minds are stuck in this way of thinking are unable to progress. They are the prisoners of their own beliefs.

Here is a simple example of the tension which exists between relying on what we know and our need to explore and challenge our skills and abilities and thereby make progress in any endeavor we undertake. Let's say that your friend has taught you to play catch with a baseball. The two of you can toss it back and forth freely with differing degrees of force and direction. Each of you easily adapts to those changes without needing to give much thought to what you are doing. You just play catch.

Now, imagine that instead of a baseball your friend unexpectedly tosses you a chunk of tofu or a raw egg. Tofu is soft and easily breaks apart. A raw egg is easily broken and then it makes an unpleasant, sticky mess. Suddenly you need to know how to catch a new material in a new way. Your mindset needs to immediately change. What you had been doing will no longer work under these new conditions. To make a successful catch you need to disregard or at least modify your old skills and abilities and progress on to something new. So, be open and prepared to catch a new idea when it appears. Learn to catch tofu.

Being a prisoner of one's own beliefs can certainly occur in tai chi. It is a well-known maxim of tai chi that "the mind moves the chi and the chi moves the body". If the mind is restricted by the limitations placed on it by its owner, then the power of the mind will be limited in what it can accomplish. Such a mindset is like a hobbled horse that is unable to run or a bird with clipped wings, unable to fly.

• *Some Further Comments on Taoist Thought:* In Taoist philosophy, there are several levels of metaphysical development. The first is the Chi (vital energy) level, the next highest is the *Yi* (mind/intent) level and the highest level is the Shen (spirit level). The limits of the mind's powers and its interactions with our bodies are not fully understood even today. Each week seems to bring with it another interesting scientific study that announces new findings regarding those body/mind interactions. Now and then such discoveries are accidental and the scientists are amazed by the unexpected results.

• *Karma & Empty Force:* In my tai chi life I have always sought out new challenges. I did not want to be bored or come to a standstill. I needed new goals, something more to achieve.

After doing "Search Center" work for several years, I decided that the next challenge would be to see if I could obtain similar results but without physically touching my partner. I originally got this idea from a story told by my I-Chuan teacher, Master Do, Tsu Jung. The story was about his own Master's bout with the Japanese soldier. When that soldier attacked the Master, the soldier was simply tossed out and flew away. This was the result of the Master's use of "Ling Kong Jin", the so-called "Empty Force". (See Chapter 4, "The I-Chuan Master".)

From Master Do, I had learned that you could develop your internal chi by doing a lot of standing posture meditation. Just by focusing your thinking, you could develop your chi. The slogan for such work was: *"Yong Yi, Bu Yong Li."* (Use the mind, not force.).

So, I set out to do this. It was an exploratory adventure. I did not know if I would succeed or fail.

From my initial "Search Center" point of contact with my partner, my method was to get a light "search" going. I then increased my mental focus on this point of contact and its relationship to my partner's center. As my mental focus improved and became stronger and stronger (Yang), I trained my physical body to relax more and remain soft (Yin) all the while. By practicing in this manner over a long period, I gradually found that the internal energy in my body was able to emerge and have a direct effect on my partner.

One day, during a "Search Center" session with a student, quite by accident my hand did not touch him but he collapsed on the bench anyway. I was certainly surprised and so was he. Something novel had occurred. In retrospect, it was an occasion of the right time, right person, and the right situation. After class, I contacted Master Do to talk to him about my experience because he had previously given a demonstration of causing a similar "No-Touch" fall in one of his pupils.

Before that event with my student, I had never had the experience of receiving or sending this empty force. I had only read about it in books or had listened to my teachers talk about it. I had always been very curious about whether or not it was real. Given what happened with my student that day, I decided to challenge myself to see if I could further develop this ability.

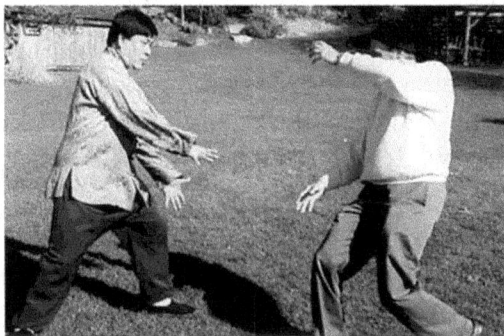

Master Wang & Joe Zanbilowicz

My new goal was to focus all my concentration on the internal feeling of the chi trail while doing my tai chi form and partner work. When I first began concentrating in this manner, I found that I would be completely exhausted, both physically and mentally, after perhaps only ten to twenty minutes of practice. This was very surprising to me because I had been involved in athletics for many years and was in very good physical condition. But after about a year or two of this type of practice, I became accustomed to it and was no longer fatigued.

The most difficult part of this manner of training is to keep your mind intensely focused (*Yang*) while your body remains entirely soft (*Yin*). If the intensity of the mental concentration slips over into a manifestation of tension in the physical body, then the physical body will become Yang at the same time the mind is already Yang. If both the mind and the body are simultaneously Yang then this method simply will not work. The internal energy is unable to flow.

I began privately practicing this empty force method with two of my senior students. As I became softer and my energy became more focused, I found that I was becoming less reliant on physical touch to move someone. We practiced in private for a couple of years until I found it could work. Then I began teaching it to my advanced students.

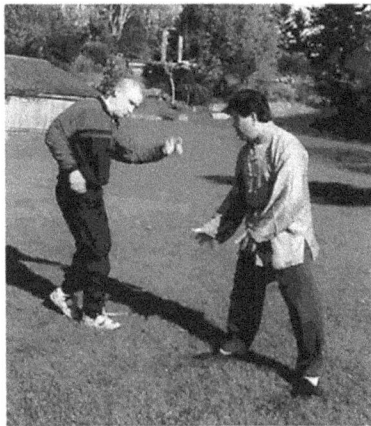

Master Wang & James Milne

Over the past few years, I have devoted countless hours of practice and research to this ability. As a result, I am now able to move many of my students without any physical contact between us. Today, I strongly believe in the capacity of a person to transmit chi over a distance and in a manner that can cause a physical reaction or effect on another person. I call this uncommon ability "No-Touch".

"No-Touch" is an outgrowth of "Search Center" that is hard to describe. I sometimes also call it "magnet power" or "wave power". However, the use of "No-Touch" does not involve the use of physical strength or power. It just destroys an opponent's Center which in turn compromises his or her balance and thereby restricts his or her ability to act. It is not brutal like other martial arts can be. For quite a few years now, I have used it successfully on both highly skilled hard-style and soft-style martial artists. These are people who have studied their particular styles for many years and are not my students. When asked about these encounters they usually can't describe exactly what occurred. The comments are generally something like this, "I don't know what happened. My body felt vulnerable but I did not feel pain or damage. I just couldn't continue my efforts to make contact with you."

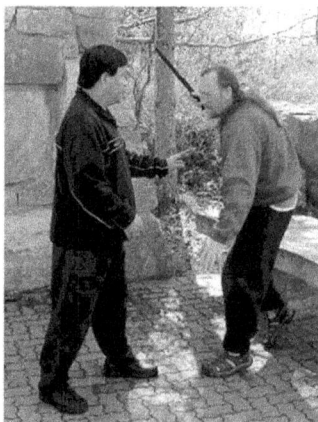

Implement in Hand
Master Wang & Greg Harley

"No-Touch" is not an idea that is suitable for people who are beginners in tai chi practice. "No-Touch" is at the Shen level, the spirit level. You will not be able to do this if you are just starting on your tai chi journey. This ability can only be achieved after years of practice and only after you have progressed through all the various preceding stages of development. There are no shortcuts. You must do the work and, most importantly, it must be the right kind of work.

Now, over thirty years later, most of my advanced students can understand the idea of the use of "No-Touch" energy. Other people still don't think it is real. I tell my students that sometimes the timing isn't right for the acceptance of new ideas. Eventually, people will get it.

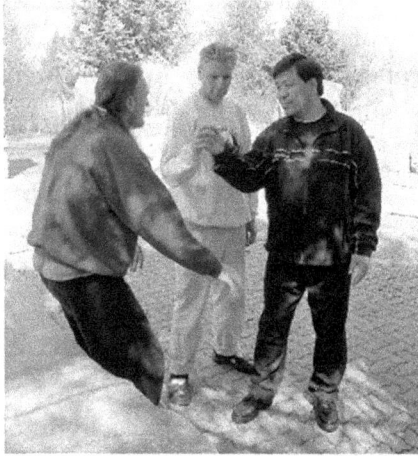

"No Touch" via Third Person
Master Wang Searches Greg Harley

• *Skeptical Concerns About Cooperation:* Other tai chi Masters before me have also claimed they possess "empty force" abilities that enable them to transmit chi energy over a distance and move an opponent without actually touching him or her. Skeptics doubt the existence of such chi transmission and claim that any reactions on the receiver's part are due to cooperation between teacher and student. They feel the student is pressured to respond as his or her master wishes; and, in turn, the master is then deluded or misled into thinking he or she has special powers.

This issue of cooperation is a difficult one to resolve. My students have reported different reactions after working with me in a "No-Touch" session. Some are extremely sensitive to this energy and fall over when I work with them. Others feel little and cannot understand why their peers are responding in such a manner when they do not. One possible explanation is that, just as I have developed certain transmission skills, those affected have themselves developed better *ting jin* (listening energy) and thus possess a heightened sensitivity to this energy.

What is the experience of "No-Touch" like for my students? They tell me that the feeling is usually quite subtle in the beginning. Over time, stronger reactions are felt. Their sensations vary. Some students are aware of a sensation of pressure. Others feel an electrical jolt. Still others report a disruption in their intentions such that they find themselves suddenly stopped in the performance of their planned actions.

My students say that they can choose to be insensitive and not respond to my "No-Touch" energy. It is possible to resist it. But there is no point in such an attitude. The purpose of tai chi is to increase our body awareness and sensitivity, develop our chi energy, and improve our health.

In practicing "Search Center", one has to become softer and learn listening skills. The use of no more than a light touch during physical contact requires the development of a heightened degree of sensitivity and relaxation. If you are too hard, it is easy for your partner to find your Center and you will be unable to find your partner's. If nothing else, the "No-Touch" work we do is an excellent exercise for developing listening skills and sensitivity. If one can detect and respond to a lack of touch, then one is more able to feel even very soft contact.

As it is a whole-body sensation and an experiential feeling, this method is very difficult to explain or satisfactorily convey in words. It is like tasting the difference between a Pu-erh tea and a high mountain oolong. If you have never tasted either, how would you know that the different characteristics I am describing for each tea are true? How do you know if my recitation of their qualities is correct?

You have to have those kinds of "No-Touch" experiences and feelings yourself. It is similar to a tea tasting. How can you judge which one is good and which one is even better? You need to drink them.

To work toward "No-Touch" you must first do "Search Center". From doing "Search Center" practice you will learn the meaning of the internal spiral and come to understand your body's internal spiral. A thorough understanding of the internal spiral is an essential prerequisite if you hope to attain "No-Touch" abilities.

• *Current Limits to This Phenomenon:* Am I able to direct this "No-Touch" energy at an unwilling or unaware person and make them move? No. At least not yet. Perhaps this is a future possibility. I feel the mind is capable of almost anything. It may only be a lack of insight or inspiration in our practice that keeps us from accomplishing what is now considered impossible.

• *Tai Chi's Benefits for Your Spirit:* In the future, I believe that "No-Touch" can become something beyond an advanced component of tai chi's martial arts skills. It is not just a physical exercise it is a Shen level practice.

In Taoism and Traditional Chinese Medicine (TCM) three essential energies support life: Jing, Chi, and Shen. In TCM they are often called "The Three Treasures" and are translated as "essence, vitality, and spirit". Jing is associated with our physical body. Chi is the life-force energy that animates our body. Shen is our spirit in the largest sense. Shen has been compared to the radiance given off by a candle flame. Chi is the flame itself. Jing is the candle's wax and wick from which the Chi emerges.

In TCM the Shen energy is the energy of the heart and is linked with the fundamental element of fire. Shen is the spirit/mind level that connects to the Tao and energizes our chi. It is the highest energy and it influences and helps calm and balance the mind and emotions. It preserves balance within ourselves. A person with a balanced Shen can follow nature's laws and universal rhythms.

As we age our physical abilities most certainly decline but if our minds can reach this Shen level then we can begin to use it. This is done by using our mental powers, not physical powers. It can become a way to prolong a healthy life through the development of a more positive outlook and an optimistic spirit. I have known people who are one hundred years old and who have gone ten or more years without doing a physical exercise routine yet continue to maintain good health. They remain well because their mental health leads their lives.

In the long run, we practice tai chi to maintain our health, to further our longevity, and to rejuvenate ourselves. "No-Touch" training operates at the Shen level and helps us eliminate negative thinking and replace it with positive thoughts that will in turn promote and help us maintain long, healthy lives. That is why I advocate and promote the spiritual aspects and potentials of tai chi over the mere physical exercise side of the art.

Tai chi will strengthen and balance Shen. With a healthy Shen, there is a feeling of inner peace and joy.

◆ ◆ ◆

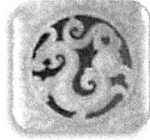

Chapter 15: Push Hands & The Soft Way

IN THE PUSH HANDS matches fought at today's tai chi tournaments around the world there is one major error repeatedly evident, the unjustifiable use of physical force *(Li)*. My use of "fought" is not a casual choice of words. I selected it deliberately because for far too long that is what seems to be occurring at these competitions - a fight. These bouts regularly feature overwhelming bursts of excessive, near frantic force. Force, coupled with occasional grappling and grasping, that only serves to further provoke and worsen the already overly aggressive mix. This is regrettable.

You might well be confused that I disapprove of fights occurring at a martial arts tournament. After all, tai chi is a martial art, and aren't the martial arts intended to equip a person with the necessary skills for self-defense in a fight? Isn't the purpose of these matches to test those very same self-defense skills? What is the problem?

It is certainly true that tai chi is a potent martial art and that these tournaments are a testing ground and measurement of the participant's skills. However, the major error I wish to discuss in this chapter is the breakdown between the gentle and soft attributes cultivated in tai chi form practice and the actual methods used in Push Hands contests. Push Hands competitions are simply not conducted in a manner that is either soft or consistent with tai chi's philosophy and principles. To confirm this yourself, you need only look at a random selection from the vast numbers of tournament video clips available on the internet. There is little softness evident in those Push Hands matches. Instead, what is seen is the use of muscular strength *(Li)*, speed, and cunning fighting techniques.

What is even more troubling, for the participants themselves and the art of tai chi, is that such tactics are being whole-heartedly encouraged by the tournament's rules. These errors of forcefulness continue to occur because acting in such a manner is rewarded by the granting of points. The current method of competition scoring has led to an obvious abandonment of tai chi's underlying philosophy of soft overcoming hard. It has also brought about a sad diminishment of the high standards which the art demands and which all practitioners should be striving to personify.

I've spent more than forty-five years practicing tai chi and observing and engaging with other martial artists from a wide variety of different martial arts disciplines other than tai chi. All those other martial arts usually depend on the use of speed and strength in utilizing the techniques and methods of their style. None of those martial arts encourage their stylists to become soft. It is only the internal style arts such as Hsing-I, Bagua, and Tai Chi Chuan that follow the soft approach, and perhaps none more so than tai chi. Unfortunately, the conduct displayed by most contemporary Push Hands contestants resembles that of the hardstyle arts instead.

• *More of the Same:* To be fair, I think that this is not just a contemporary phenomenon. I think it is an old and recurring problem for all tai chi players. I competed in tai chi Push Hands tournaments for ten years in Taiwan and was a champion five times. So, I am speaking from my own experience and from the experience of those I have encountered along the way.

In my tai chi career, I was fortunate to have been well-schooled in the philosophy and ideals of tai chi and always sought to incorporate those concepts in my form practice. When I began to participate in Push Hands competitions, I resolved to try to use the soft skills related to sensation and root in those circumstances as well. But, when faced with an adversary, I soon discarded the ideals I used

246

in my form practice and began acting mistakenly during tournament matches.

In my matches, I used a 70/30 front foot posture and often relied on speed, technique, and physical strength in pushing my opponent. Indeed, all of us who competed at that time were training and acting in this fashion. This was simply how the competition was done in those days and unfortunately, that type of behavior is still largely the case today.

At the time, I thought I was doing what was expected, appropriate, and even required of a tai chi competitor. However, my behavior was not true tai chi. Only in later years did I understand that what I had been doing was incorrect. Incorrect because it was not based on tai chi philosophy and the principles normally embraced while engaged in the practice of the tai chi form.

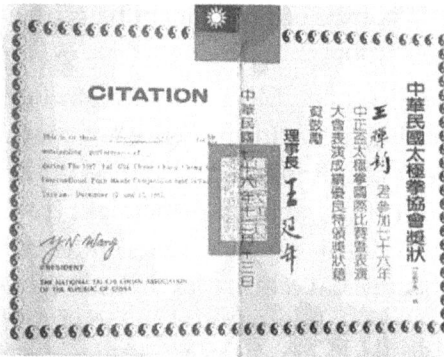

Certificate Awarded to Master Wang
The National Tai Chi Chuan Association of the Republic of China
December 1987

• *Like a Three-Legged Stool:* In tai chi today, and most likely in earlier periods in tai chi history as well, there is a widespread lack of harmony among its three principal elements. The first element is the underlying theory and tai chi philosophy. Second, there is tai chi form practice. The third part is the applied use of tai chi postures either in Push Hands competitions or in martial arts applications. Although the pieces of this trio are all interrelated and should be joined together, in the real world they often are not. Whether by intention or, as is more likely, out of ignorance and misunderstanding, they are and remain disconnected. Each is pursued separately and without a full appreciation of the important need to both recognize and develop their underlying unity.

These three components are like the supports of a three-legged stool. Remove any one leg and the stool no longer functions according to its nature. The purpose for which it was intended can no longer be fulfilled. The now faulty seat becomes not only useless, but it is also pointless as well. Similarly, if the tai chi philosophical principles cultivated in form practice are abandoned during competition situations then competitive tai chi is being done in a manner that is no longer true to its nature. The same conclusion would also apply if the principles are discarded in the heat of a full-blown, self-defense situation. In either case, the activities engaged in by the participants are no longer genuine tai chi and instead become something else. This type of false tai chi has come to be as pointless as that two-legged stool.

• *The Typical Situation:* Most students start on their tai chi path by taking a beginning tai chi form class. They may also read about tai chi history and philosophy and gain a certain intellectual understanding of its fundamental principles. They then begin to pay more attention to form practice and endeavor to embody the principles which they have heard and read. While this is a correct approach, they soon begin to struggle as they find that their bodies do not readily accept or easily adopt the traits that their minds command. There is a gap between their intentions and their ability to execute those intended actions appropriately. They find that it is not easy to express or exemplify something so abstract and intangible while engaged in the concrete, physical act of tai chi form practice. Even so, as they do the necessary work, they at least strive to be quiet, soft, and relaxed in the performance of the form. Eventually, they will succeed in learning the entire sequence of postures which their style of tai chi contains.

Next, they may engage in Push Hands practice during class or perhaps even join Push Hands competitions. Sadly, in those classroom practice situations, and even more often in tournaments, they quickly return to the use of tremendous physical strength while they thrash about with each other. At the outset of these encounters, you can clearly see that the contestant's main attitude toward each other is one of confrontation and opposition. Particularly in tournaments, the participants are immediately at odds and even openly hostile toward each other. By behaving in this antagonistic and often aggressive manner, they display the lack of anything related to tai chi theory or tai chi philosophy. The softness and relaxation associated with their tai chi form practice are likewise abandoned. They don't remember the classic tai chi instruction that it is necessary to invest in loss. They fail to recall that to succeed at developing tai chi skills one must give up the self and ambition and instead learn to be neutral and to follow the lead of the other person.

• *Correct Logic but Mistaken Idea:* Some years ago, our tai chi group participated in a tai chi tournament and Push Hands competition in Vancouver, British Columbia. A local tai chi organization invited us. We had the largest group of people entered. I accepted their kind invitation because I hoped to show the other tai chi groups my "Search Center" idea about how competitions should be conducted. I wanted to demonstrate our group's thinking about how to proceed in a soft way during Push Hands matches.

In talking to my students who were going to compete, I told them just to see how confident they could be in performing their tai chi form or doing Push Hands in such a public setting. I told them not to think about doing Push Hands in the usual manner because in the typical tournament situation, even at the highest level, it still involved speed, technique, and strength. Those elements are the same ones common to many other martial arts. They are not the unique traits that separate tai chi from those other martial arts.

I told them that the point of having them compete was not that they should win the trophy. The point was to have them develop a relaxed, calm, self-assured, and composed presentation in the face of this public scrutiny and judgment. Their level of composure and self-confidence was something they could judge for themselves.

A telling and rather significant incident occurred during that weekend. One of the judges took me aside to talk to me about my students' behavior. He said that although the contestants from our school were very good, they did not know how to push! He proposed that I should teach my students to fight. Initially, I was inwardly amused and somewhat startled by his well-intentioned advice. Afterward, I came to believe that this judge did not have a complete understanding of the philosophy behind the art. If he did, he would have realized that when you successfully yield to an incoming push the Yin/negative power displayed while yielding is necessarily equivalent to the amount of the Yang/positive power of the incoming push. If you are pushed and can respond with a matching yield, the result will be neutral. If it isn't, you will be thrown out. I think he did not see or appreciate this point. The power demonstrated via a timely and successful neutralization is equivalent in such circumstances.

One reason he overlooked this neutralization equivalence was due to the tournament organizers' preexisting judgments about what the scoring rules for the competition should be. No matter how well-intentioned, the rule-makers themselves did not realize that their rules ran counter to the underlying principles of the tai chi art. The rules were set up so that only the one who pushes more effectively is declared the winner. It was not possible to score any points for a yield that effectively neutralized an incoming push.

During that competition, and in other competitions in subsequent years that we attended, it was only our group that worked in the soft way. We only sought to be soft, yield, control the partner's center, and not push with physical force. Perhaps not surprisingly, our group was repeatedly criticized for being too soft and for not pushing. Everyone else wondered why we behaved in this manner. They could not understand it. It was thought that we did not have any power in our tai chi. For five years we went to the Vancouver tournament and other competitions as well but my "Search Center" idea never caught on. I couldn't influence them to adopt this far less aggressive approach. So, after devoting all that time to working our tai chi in this soft way, our group decided that we should just stop going to tournaments.

At those competitions and even thereafter, I always invited peopled to come to the Comox Elementary School for our Sunday morning, "Search Center" practice; but, no one from outside our group ever came. Through the years we've simply continued with our practice. Perhaps others will come to visit eventually.

• *An Outsider Provides a Lesson:* Sometimes people who study judo or wrestling come to watch these Push Hands competitions and they often remark that what they are witnessing would not be difficult for them to do. They think that they could win this type of competition. Indeed, one of my senior students recently reminded me of just such a competition held many years ago at Capilano University in North Vancouver. A gentleman who had never studied tai chi entered the tournament. He had studied karate and had participated in karate competitions. He walked in, shoved his opponent, and walked out with the trophy. He knew nothing about tai chi.

• *The Unsuitable Current Rules:* As a former champion, I know well the trouble with the current system. To win, you must be able to push successfully. You can only score points on offense, not on defense. Competitors realize this; and, in their eagerness to win, they quickly give up the characteristics and principles contained in the tai chi form. The tai chi on display then becomes very low quality.

Indeed, as a result of some mistaken notions about the true nature of the soft style arts, some tournaments are now requiring that helmets be worn for the safety of the competitors. Of course, safety is always important. But, helmets! Imagine that. There is no soft benefit there. There is no soft result. When it comes to competitive events, everyone, including competitors and judges, quickly forgets what they are supposed to be studying. They are not devoted to putting the idea of the soft way into practical use.

The current obsession with comparing the hand-to-hand fighting aspects of tai chi applications to those of other martial arts, including mixed martial arts (MMA) matches, is counter to the basic tenets of Taoist philosophy. People who are so narrowly focused on the brutal competitive aspects such as those displayed during MMA matches lose sight of tai chi's many health-related benefits. Such a focus distorts the broader assortment of rewards tai chi offers and is not only philosophically wrong but ultimately also self-defeating.

All games follow a set of rules but the object of each game may be quite different. In basketball, you can only use your hands to move the ball and score. In soccer, it is just the opposite. You primarily use your feet to score and the hands must never be used. In basketball, the more points you make the better because the higher score wins. However, if you play golf, it's just the opposite. The winner is the player with the lowest score.

So, why is it that in tai chi tournaments you can only score points by making a successful push? Why are points not given for yielding, neutralizing, and/or avoiding a push? Tournament scoring can certainly be calculated in other ways that are more conducive to producing players who correctly embody the highest principles of the art of tai chi. Even in China and Taiwan people are still thinking about these things in the wrong way.

Outside of competitive tournaments, traditional tai chi instruction puts great emphasis on developing a soft form and slow, graceful movements. The student is encouraged to flow like water and to move in harmony with nature's way. The tai chi ideal should be to treat your Push Hands partner in the same soft way and utilize the principles of Yin and Yang in response to an opponent's aggression. Aggression and force should not be countered with aggression and force.

For example, in fixed-step matches, instead of attacking and pushing back in response to an opponent's push, you should conceptually "step back" and thereby yield. I do not mean to move your feet during a fixed-step match. I mean that your first response should be to yield and neutralize. You should learn to relax, accept, and neutralize the incoming force. Not resist. Not clash. Not act in muscular opposition to your partner's force and intention. As participants, you don't want to act like two bulls fighting or two rams butting heads. Advancement of the tai chi art requires more appropriate rules.

• *Rethinking the Current Rules:* In all types of traditional martial arts competitions, the person who delivers the decisive, debilitating blows or throws his or her opponent out is the person who scores the point and eventually wins the match. In traditional martial arts competitions, the rewards and honors go to the fastest, strongest, and most powerful competitors. The result, even where the stated goal is not to injure or disable the opponent, is that the opponents are often injured, sometimes seriously.

The time for these traditional ideas in competitive martial arts has largely passed. For the vast majority of today's martial arts programs, the purpose of participation is to improve one's health, to benefit the body, and to enjoy the society and companionship of like-minded people who share an interest in the art. The purpose is not to see the opponent fearful, bleeding, hurt, or otherwise injured.

I believe that the time is now right for a revolutionary change in how all martial arts, not just tai chi, but all hard and soft styles of fighting, are viewed.

For this to happen, there must first be an open inquiry into the philosophy on which the art is based. As explained in Lao Tse's philosophy, Taoist cosmology maintains that the myriad items that come into and go out of existence ("the ten thousand things") emerge from the creative power of the undifferentiated emptiness/one known as Wu Chi (Wuji/unity). Wu Chi is depicted as an empty circle and implies a Tao of non-duality. From this void of non-duality, the simultaneous differentiation into Yin and Yang occurs and all the phenomena of the observable world are subsequently and consequentially produced. The familiar tai chi or Yin/Yang symbol depicts that manifestation. This original creative power comes from nothing. This power comes from softness.

I developed my idea for the "Search Center" practice method in response to and in furtherance of those philosophical principles. Those who are engaged in the practice of "Search Center" are immersed in developing the idea of emptiness and cultivating the sensation and use of the chi flow which is occurring within and between them. The paired partners are engaged in a different and I think more enjoyable type of martial arts contest. It is a contest to see who can be soft, who can yield, who can put Lao Tse's philosophy into practice in the real world. They want to see and learn if and how it is possible, through the use of the internal chi, to develop power without needing to use physical strength. "Search Center" matches would still be a contest but one with a different purpose and approach. And, at the highest level, "Search Center" is also an extremely effective method of self-defense that need not cause injury or trauma to the opponent yet can protect the practitioner.

Regrettably, although tai chi philosophy emphasizes softness and relaxation, the rules of Push Hands competitions do not follow those principles. As previously mentioned, in traditional Push Hands tournaments, if you push the other person you can win a point. But if you are soft, relaxed, and yielding you do not win points for those significant accomplishments. If you neutralize or yield to a push you do not get a point. If pushing is the only type of conduct that is rewarded under the rules, I wonder where the incentive is to cultivate a soft way of practice. Why would competitors need to develop a soft way of practice? Why would people even need to think about a philosophy which talks about the soft way as being in the end the source of real power? The use of physical force which the current rules encourage and reward is an idea that is totally against tai chi principles and tai chi form practice. Such rules merely pit one person against another as an obstacle to be overcome.

All of this discussion is perhaps familiar territory to anyone who has been practicing tai chi for a few years. The larger point I'm trying to make here is that a major reason for this disharmony can be directly traced back to the rules which are set up for these Push Hands competitions. The rules necessarily provide some safe boundaries as to what is allowed as acceptable conduct but they also provide the exclusive method for determining who is the winner. However, if these rules are themselves developed from faulty premises you will necessarily end up with faulty outcomes.

The "Search Center" training method I have developed can become the new approach for improving what occurs during a Push Hands competition. I believe it would be a change for the better since it will re-link tai chi's underlying Taoist philosophy with actual competitive practice. In "Search Center" practice the sensation of the contact at the moment of touching hands with your partner is used to judge your partner's force and to find his "stuck point". A person skilled in this method is then able to move his opponent using internal energy and very little physical movement.

• *My Rules Change Proposal:* It is my firm conviction that there is a way to improve tai chi competition that would make it compatible with the underlying philosophy of tai chi. The solution to this problem should start by making changes in how these contests are scored and judged.

I'd like to see the rules for Push Hands tournaments changed to give proper recognition for the skillful use of tai chi's soft way. I would change the rules to award points to the player who can remain soft and yielding in response to the opponent's physical push. If you use physical force to push, no point should be given. If you lose your center while pushing, no point is scored. If you neutralize, you get a point. If you yield, you get a point. So, if you want to solve this problem, I think the rules of competition should be changed in this way. Push Hands matches should never be fights.

Here is what I propose. In the future, Push Hands competitions should consist of two rounds. During the first round, one person would be designated as the Searcher/Sender (offense) and the other the Searchee/Receiver (defense). During the second round, the roles would be reversed. By establishing these two different roles for the participants each gains the benefit of seeing both sides of the coin, the Yin and Yang aspects of interacting with your partner. Learning to balance the requirements of both modes of interaction is the most harmonious way to practice. Additionally, under this system, it is not just the Yang side that can score points as is now the case. If my proposal is adopted the Yin side can also score points.

This contest will require two judges for each match. One to watch and score the Searcher/Sender. The other to watch and score the Searchee/Receiver.

The match will last a total of six minutes. There will be two, three-minute rounds and the Searcher/Searchee roles will alternate. Scoring would be done during each of the unlimited numbers of search events which the Searcher is allowed to make during a three-minute round. All searches must be initiated by the Searcher. The Searcher would endeavor to use "Search Center" principles to score points. The encounter is about sensation. The Searcher/Sender's task is to discover where his or her partner is stuck and unable to yield. This is done through the use of one's lightest touch to determine the partners' degree of muscular forcefulness, resistance, and bodily tension. The goal is to lock onto the Searchee/Receiver's center in such a manner that he or she will not have a chance to avoid and yield to the search. Description of this activity in words is hard to convey but is readily understood when engaged with an experienced player.

If the scorekeeping rules of the contest are changed in this way the combative attitude which is so predominant today will change for the better. By proceeding in this manner, the participants will get the true benefits of soft practice. Also, I believe that more women will participate because they will find that it is a more agreeable way to practice since the use of aggressive and forceful means is not rewarded. Skill is required; not dull force.

The simultaneous scoring would follow these rules:

On the Searcher/Sender's Side: Offense

1. If you search outside the centerline and try for a lock but your center leans; you will lose a point.

2. If you search for the center and physically push, you will lose a point.

3. If you search and try for a hard lock utilizing a physical grab of your partner, you will lose a point.

4. If you search and try for a lock but come out of your root, you will lose a point.

5. If you search and can lock an opponent, without incurring any of the four violations, you score a point. If the

256

Searcher over-leans, or uses strength, or pushes, or is out of his/her center then no point is scored.

On the Searchee/Receiver's Side: Defense

1. If you try to avoid the search by yielding but lose your root, you will lose a point.

2. If you try to yield by randomly moving your body without first sensing and responding to the incoming search, you will lose a point.

3. If you yield and avoid a lock, without incurring either of the two violations, you score a point,

4. If you yield using a small circle and internal spiral you will win the point. If you yield by just releasing your arm you will not win a point.

The person with the higher number of points after the two rounds wins the match.

• *Contrasting Viewpoints in Martial Arts:* "Search Center" is a more difficult, challenging, and complex way toward progress in the martial arts. Perhaps no greater contrast could be found to its methods than the methods on display in the currently popular mixed martial arts (MMA) fighting competitions. Contests of that nature are truly bouts of brutality. The participants are expected to fight until their opponents are injured so severely that he or she either can't respond or is otherwise rendered unable to further defend themselves. It is based on an ugly premise because it encourages people to behave savagely against one another. Its nearly unrestrained violence offers little or no spiritual benefit to either competitor. Many people like to watch MMA but it is like watching a dog fight or cockfight. It appeals to our baser nature.

By way of contrast, Aikido is one example of martial arts that is not like that at all. Its philosophy is more advanced. There is never an aikido competition. There are only aikido demonstrations. It is an art meant for self-defense; but, at the same time, it does not require inflicting incapacitating injury upon the aggressor. Those who practice aikido do not fight among themselves and they do not fight against students of other martial arts. This attitude is good; it is more spiritual.

• *My Promotion of the "Search Center" Idea:* I was fortunate in my life to have met Master Huang, Sheng Shyan. Had I not encountered him I think that I would still be doing Push Hands in my earlier, mistaken manner. I would not have realized my error and not found the correct path. Had he not come to Taiwan to give a demonstration and had I not taken that first opportunity to observe him in person, my tai chi life would have been completely different. In my mind, that initial meeting and all that followed from it is karma.

Now, I want to develop and share this knowledge that I have since gained. I feel it is important to tell the people in the world who are doing tai chi that they should not follow the old method and style of doing Push Hands. Instead, they need to remember tai chi principles. They need to do competitive tai chi in a manner that is only principle-based. Partner work done in the "Search Center" manner embodies those principles and with sufficient practice becomes a very powerful martial art. It epitomizes the soft way.

• *A New Idea Takes Time:* I live in Canada and have traveled to Europe, the United States, Asia, and Taiwan to give workshops. I find that people are not yet receptive to this message. It is very difficult for them to understand the significance of what I am advocating. Although they have seen me give convincing demonstrations of its effectiveness, they do not understand how I can do what I do. So, that's why I have written this book. The message is hard for people to understand. It is hard to get people to realize just how different my training method is and what it asks of people. It is not something they are familiar with so they don't immediately understand how much it can benefit them.

That's why I promote my ideas about tai chi. I seek to develop a wider audience and awareness of a particular idea by talking about it at workshops. My ideas about tai chi have been developed gradually over more than forty-five years of intense study and practice. In my development of these concepts, I have been fortunate to have been associated with and learned a great deal from many tai chi masters. Through them and with my subsequent efforts and experimentation, I believe that I have been able to find the best course for the evolution and future advancement of tai chi for the next generation.

From personal experience, I know what results from training in the old-style Push Hands methods and practices. In that type of Push Hands work you make people tense, you make people angry, you make people frustrated. Sometimes, you make people frightened. That's why lots of people choose to just do the tai chi form and are not interested in Push Hands.

If the approach to Push Hands work is switched to my "Search Center" method there is no violence. There is only sensation, there is only touch hands, there is just search your center. Once exposed to this method of interaction, I believe many more people will become very interested in this type of partner practice. You set up a new series of rules. If there is no benefit to be gained from a physical push the participants will now think about the benefit to be realized from the soft way, the tai chi way.

In my workshops, I practice with many different people of all ages, backgrounds, and skill levels. Never has a person been hurt or gotten angry. Along with a seriousness of purpose about the practice, there is always laughter in the room. When you see this kind of feeling and attitude occurring between tai chi partners, that's what I'm talking about.

• *Time for a Name Change?* My adult life has been devoted to the study and practice of the Chinese martial art "Tai Chi Chuan" (Taijiquan), an art that developed out of the practical need for an effective method of self-defense to defeat an attacker. It is a fighting art. Its very name proclaims it as the best of such arts, the "Supreme Ultimate Fist". When utilized by a skilled practitioner it is indeed a highly effective method of self-defense.

I now think that for the next generation, for those who follow after me, the name of this art should be changed to reflect an emphasis on the study of tai chi as a practice that entails more than just a fighting art. At the highest levels, tai chi is a philosophy, a

259

method to improve one's health, an activity that promotes camaraderie and friendships, and a method of non-violent yet powerful martial art. Its depths can be studied throughout one's life without ever being exhausted. Consequently, I think that for the future the more appropriate term for this study is "Tai Chi Dao" rather than "Tai Chi Chuan". This phrase more accurately indicates that the study of the art of tai chi is a pathway that can be followed for one's entire life.

I also think that partner practice in tai chi should no longer be called Push Hands. The name for this activity should be changed to "touch hands" or "sensation hands". The purpose of this change is to reflect a more fruitful and mutually beneficial way of conducting tai chi partner practice. The object of this type of practice is to become aware of your center and at the same time to find and control the other person's center. That's why I use the term "Search Center" rather than Push Hands and propose that others use it as well.

• *Developing a Posture's Proper Shape is Key:* When teaching tai chi, putting the focus or emphasis on the martial arts function of a particular posture is not the best way to develop one's internal energy power. Emphasis on composing a proper position and shape is the most important aspect of worthwhile instruction when learning any particular tai chi posture, regardless of the style being studied. For example, in most tai chi classes today, when teaching the posture "Push" (*An*), the shape of the arms and body are arranged in a manner that suggests and encourages both the thought and the action of pushing or shoving someone. To focus on the verb "push" is to put the idea into the student's head that the proper result will only come from the use of muscular strength (*Li*). But, in truth, when performing any posture, the proper effect comes from the use of tai chi's internal power (*nei jin*) not from the use of physical strength (*Li*). Such power is possible only if the shape of each posture is correctly composed and internally connected. No importance or instruction needs to be given concerning the action of pushing.

Such internal power (*nei jin*) is best developed by training the entire body to become coordinated and internally connected while executing the movements necessary to achieve the proper balanced and proportionate shape of the posture. The appropriate instructional emphasis is to place the student's attention on the development of the correct shape of the posture being studied. Composing the proper shape allows the joints to be open and the body to be relaxed (*Sung*) in a manner that enables and facilitates the flow of the internal chi. This emphasis on "shaping" is done to enable the best possible expression and manifestation of internal energy. In the "Push" posture, the instruction is not done to promote or focus on the physical act of pushing or shoving.

However, most people studying tai chi today are stuck at the purely external level of this shape as it relates to undertaking and carrying out a physical action such as a push. At the external shape level, you can only do the physical act. You compare speed and strength. That's all people can do. You compare speed or power and whoever does that better wins. To work this way does not offer a means for attaining the highest levels which the art has to offer to those who are intensely dedicated to improving their practice.

• *Preserving the Martial Aspects of the Art:* It must always be remembered that Tai Chi Chuan is a martial art. Its development was grounded in self-defense and applied martial arts practices. Hence the name is translated as" Supreme Ultimate Fist" or "Supreme Fighting Art". But the art of tai chi is not simply limited to fighting. It is multifaceted and more profound. It also has a rich philosophy, the ability to improve and sustain one's health, and a meditative and spiritual development component as well. Since all these other attributes of the art are currently drawing the most attention, now might be the right time for a name change that better acknowledges these other inherent components of the discipline. It is time to decrease the emphasis on just the fighting aspects and to simply discontinue using the word "chuan" (fist) when referring to the art. In the future, just using the words "Tai Chi Dao" would be a sufficient and more accurate description of this truly, multi-dimensional art.

I realize that this may be considered an unorthodox and even heretical idea by those whose inclinations and preferences are to preserve the traditional aspects of this art as a fighting art.

Nevertheless, the plain truth is that those interested in tai chi as an applied fighting art are fewer and fewer in number these days. Regardless of where they live or whatever cultural background they come from, the overwhelming majority of people practicing tai chi today are attracted to it because it is reputed to help them achieve and maintain health and vitality well into old age. They simply are not interested in the martial arts potential contained within the postures of the tai chi form.

Those interested in the applied martial arts aspects of tai chi need not be concerned or alarmed that this "practical" side to the art (the original reason for its development) will be lost by this suggested name change. I am not for a moment advocating that self-defense skills not be taught. On the contrary, in "Search Center" practice lies the basis for an extremely effective method of self-defense; but, one that is harmonious in practice with the tai chi philosophy and tai chi form. Tai chi would be incomplete and a lesser art if those fighting skills were abandoned and I have absolutely no wish to see that happen. However, let there be no mistake, it takes correct instruction and diligent practice over a long time to attain the required level of skill necessary to use internal energy and not physical strength in an applied martial arts context. Faithful practice of "Search Center" principles and methods will provide the pathway to develop this martial ability but it will likely take many years of "eating bitter" before an effective demonstration of its use as a fighting art is achieved. Based on my own experience, I can assure you this is true.

> *"I consider it essential that tai chi's Taoist philosophy, tai chi form practice, and tai chi as a practical means of self-defense should all reflect a consistent point of view."*
>
> Master Henry Wang

◆ ◆ ◆

APPENDICES

◆ ◆ ◆

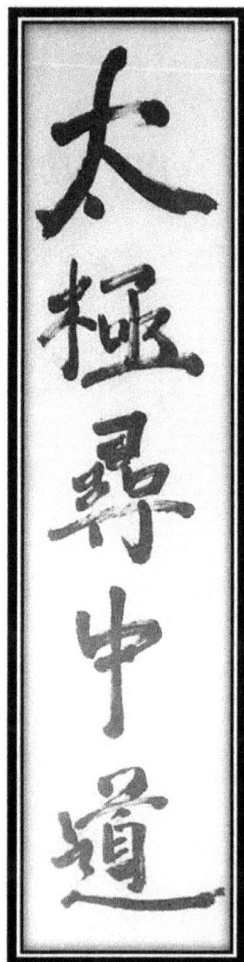

"Tai Chi Search Center Way"
Practice Studio Scroll, Comox, B.C.
Master Wang's Calligraphy

264

Appendix A: "One Hand Circling"

Spiral Energy in Partner Practice

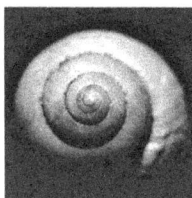

In Master Wang's classes, the students do various partner practice exercises. Some of them are "fixed-step" and others are "moving-step". One of the fixed-step drills is called "One Hand Circling".

The partners stand facing one another, each in an Archer's Stance [i.e., feet are shoulder-width apart, the front foot is advanced and pointed straight ahead and the back foot turned outward at a forty-five (45°) angle]. An imaginary line is drawn on the floor and the toes of their front feet are on either side of that line; the toes never cross over it. Their weight is equally distributed on each foot, 50/50. If the left foot is forward, they each present the back of their left hand to their partner so that the backs of their wrists are lightly touching. As a variation, they can also start by presenting the hand opposite the forward foot. Throughout the interaction the wrists remaining touching; there are no gaps or separations.

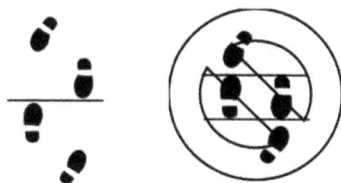

Then, by turning their Centers and using a rotation of the trunk, they proceed to circle the body and arms on a horizontal plane. As the hips turn, the *kwa* (kua) opens and closes as the trunk rotates, it is as if their forearms are smoothly gliding along a slippery tabletop. As people become more familiar with the drill, variations in the plane of movement are added. With a little practice, the interactions become more random in direction, speed, and intensity. Among other things, the partners are instructed not to provide any resistance to the incoming force and to never lose contact with each other.

Making the Spiral Occur During One Hand Circling

You begin with the central axis of your body. The central axis of your body is your Center. You can think of this axis as an imaginary straight line around which your body rotates in a balanced, proportional, and symmetrical manner.

Your weight is distributed 50/50 on each foot. Then you drop your weight into your foot at the "bubbling well" point. The foot controls both the weight of your body and the body's Center.

When you turn (rotate) the axis of the body you should notice that the pressure of the body's weight on the foot changes, even if only slightly. So, as you rotate and turn the hips and shoulders the weighted pressure will automatically be shifting from foot to foot without the necessity of moving the body from one side to the other.

Those pressure changes relate to the rotational movement of the torso/trunk around the central axis of your body. This is not an intentional shifting of weight and the body following along. For example, it is not a weight shift from one 70/30 posture to another 70/30 posture.

Instead, in my "Search Center" method, the weight of the body stays 50/50, equally distributed on each foot. You are then properly aligned with the central axis of the body and as you turn on that axis you naturally have and produce the internal spiral. Contrary to traditional doctrine, standing in this manner where you stay in your own Center, is not a "double weighted" condition. The upper body is light while the lower body is heavy and rooted. The Yin/Yang relationship between the upper and lower body averts a "double weighted" condition.

Practitioners who don't understand this idea are missing the true significance of the symbolism contained in the tai chi diagram.

In that diagram, the Yin fish (dark) has a little circle of Yang energy and the Yang fish (light) likewise contains a little circle of Yin energy. Neither is exclusively one or the other. They each contain a small element of the other. They also each join together in harmony to make the complete circle which in turn is one whole unit consisting of two symmetrical parts.

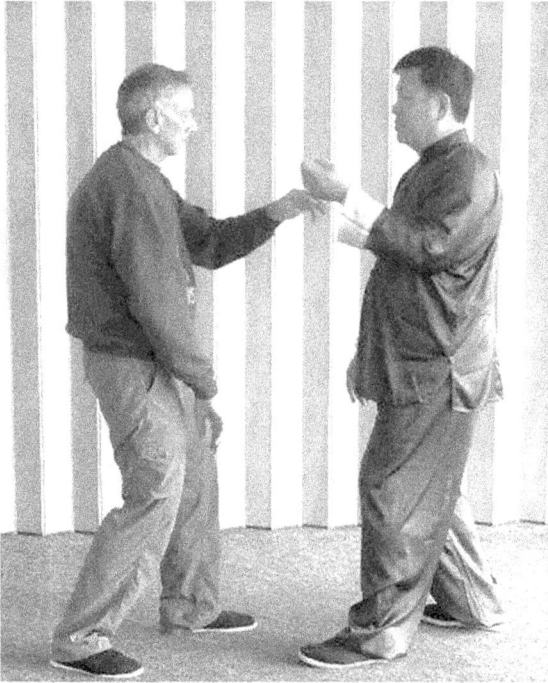

Peter Uhlmann & Master Wang

How then are we to put these ideas into practice while doing "One Hand Circling"? The spiral energy is like a lasso. You can throw that energy far away to catch your opponent. Without the spiral, you lack the lasso itself. In your form practice, if you have consistently trained properly to develop more internal spiral energy, then, when you make that initial contact with your partner, just by turning your body a little bit you can swallow a much larger incoming force. On the other hand, if you do not have this internal spiral then it will be hard to get away and you will carry more stress and tension throughout your body. It is like the principle of centrifugal force.

A centrifugal force is a force that makes an object move away from the center of something else when the object is moving around that something. A simple example is the "hammer throw" in track and field. In that event, the athlete grabs the handle of a cable which is attached to a heavy steel ball that rests on the ground. He or she extends the arms, stretches the line taut, and then begins to forcefully rotate the entire body in a series of multiple spiraling circles. The ball starts to lift off the ground and spin around with the whirling athlete like a planet orbiting the sun. Then, at the optimal moment, the grip on the handle is released so the ball and its tether can fly away on an outward seeming tangent.

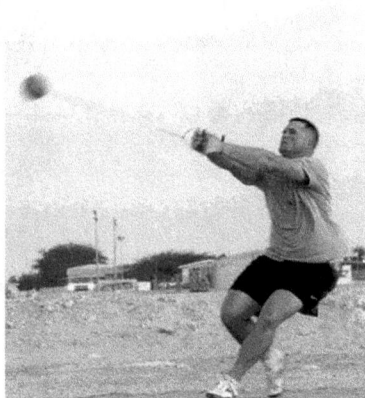

Hammer Throw Centrifugal Force

In tai chi's use of centrifugal force, a small internal turn radiates outward to cause a big effect. If your partner has the spiral energy and you don't, the further away you are from the center point of their spiraling, rotational energy the more affected you are by that energy. The more likely it is that you are going to be sent flying away. Spun off by the rotational forces spreading outward from your partner's Center.

So, as you practice your tai chi form you should strive to make spiral energy. You work and work until your entire body becomes both soft and synchronized. The left foot has the proper proportionate relationship with the right hand and vice versa. The movement of the entire body becomes harmonized in time and action. It doesn't matter how soft and relaxed you are if your movements are not also synchronized in such a manner. Achieving correct timing and arriving at the right place at the right moment is essential for the internal energy to transfer through your own body and then out of your body and directly into that of your partner.

By way of comparison, this synchronization is like twisting a wet towel to wring out the water. If the rotational, twisting pressure is not applied equally from both hands you are unable to squeeze out the unwanted water. In tai chi, that equal pressure applied uniformly from both sides is the manifestation of the spiral energy. You should work your tai chi form in this manner.

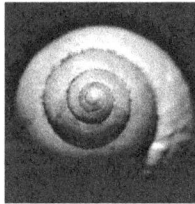

Appendix B: The Two-Fisted Pinkie Grab

A "Search Center" Exercise

This is a basic "Search Center" exercise that introduces the practical use of the "Globe Shape" in partner work. The initial positioning uses a vertical, spine-to-spine alignment. In this exercise, the players line up facing one another in an Archer's Stance. Both people have their left foot forward. Both are on the back foot (weight distribution 100/0) to start and the toes of the front foot are on either side of that "line in the sand". After the first few successful searches, the roles are switched. Both players will learn something valuable during this exercise even though one is considered receptive and the other active.

Player A's role is "active" in that she will be doing the "searching" to find Player B's center. Once found she will use her "internal energy", without physical force, to move Player B.

Player B's. role is "receptive" in that he will allow Player A to search for and find his center. He will not try to hide his center from her. If needed he will give her verbal cues about how to adjust her "search" to locate his center. When he feels Player A's energy, but not strength, extended or expanded toward him he will not resist or attempt to evade it. He will instead follow the path of that energy and allow it to push or move him in whatever direction it is going.

As a result of the exercise Player A learns: (1.) how to sense/feel whether she is in her center, (2.) how to locate and "connect" to Player B's center and what the related sensation/feeling is, (3.) how to use internal energy (*nei jin*) to move Player B without using physical force, (4.) how to initiate movement of the internal energy from her center first and not have the movement start from her hands and arms.

As a result of the exercise Player B learns: (1.) how to sense/feel whether he is in his center, (2.) what the related sensation/feeling is when someone finds his center and "connects" to it, (3.) how to read his partner's searches by sensing whether they are on or off his center and any misdirection that is taking place, (4.) how to develop a heightened sense of his center as well as that of his partner's searches by giving appropriate verbal directions to bring the "search" to his center, (5.) what the sensation of responding to internal energy feels like and how to not resist it.

Player A first puts up her hands in the "Push" posture. Keeping her arms apart, she then rotates her forearms so that the open palms are facing one another. She then makes a loose fist with both hands so the palms are closed. Next, she opens and extends only her pinkie finger on both hands while the rest of the fingers remain closed in the loose fist position. When opened, the tips of both pinkie fingers point toward Player B.

Player B does the same thing with his hands. He makes the same two loose fists but does not extend his pinkie fingers. The fists are in the same vertical orientation position they would be when completing "Parry and Punch". The thumb and forefinger face the ceiling while the closed pinkie faces the floor. The backs of the wrists face outward to the side walls while the insides of the forearms face each other.

From these two positions, we want Player B to grab Player A's extended pinkie fingers. This is done by B sliding his fist down over A's pinkie so that A's pinkie is poking up toward the top of B's fist where B's thumb and forefinger are located. The tip of A's pinkie is visible when looking down into the top of B's fist. When making each fist, Player B's fist should enclose A's pinkie fingers and he should then squeeze the pinkies firmly but not too tight and without causing any discomfort to Player A.

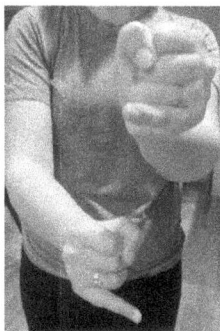

Player A Extends Fingers   *Player B Squeezes Fingers*
The joined hands are lined up on the centerline, spine to spine.

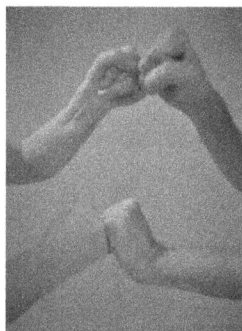

Player A should next move her hands so they are lined up on her centerline with her right hand being lower than and beneath the left. Player B should let her move his arms in this manner. In the final position, the hands of both players are aligned with their spines on the central vertical axis of their bodies.

This is now the "Start Position" for the exercise. Player A is the more "active" person in the exercise. Player B's job is to listen, comply, and not resist when Player A gets it right. Player B's job is also to help Player A find his center by giving verbal instructions if needed. These instructions will likely be needed the first few times Player A starts a search.

Remember that both people are on the back foot (weight distribution 100/0) to start. After several successful searches, Player A can also start from the 50/50 weight distribution position while Player B remains on the back foot. As experience is gained the partners can experiment with various combinations of weight distribution.

For Beginners, the exercise starts with Player B putting just a little bit of light physical force forward so that there is a "connection" established between the two players. In response, Player A does not give up any space and does not let the shape or position of her arms change. The players are just to establish a gentle "connection".

Once that is established, Player B can back off the use of physical strength slightly but must at all times maintain a "firm grip" on Player A's pinkie fingers. The firm grip is what gives Player A the chance to find and read Player B's center. A less firm grip should only be used by more advanced players.

The task is learning how to connect to your partner and use internal energy (*nei jin*) to affect their Center and disrupt their Balance without using physical force *(Li)*. Player A starts an active "search" to find Player B's center point. Once B's center point is found, Player A does not move her hands in space at all. Instead, she focuses her mind and uses her mental intention (Yi) to extend her chi energy into B's center point. Once B senses that A's energy has contacted his center, he should allow A's energy to move him in whatever direction the energy is going. B's task is to listen for and follow that energy stream.

On A's side, it is important to maintain the constant intention to move the energy until B has "fallen out". If B starts to respond to the energy, A must continue and not stop the intent. If the intent stops the energy's movement effect will also stop. On B's side if you feel the energy stop or the connection break you should stop your movement and tell A that the connection and effect have been broken.

This exercise requires a cooperative/collaborative approach. It is not a competition. For two people with no prior experience, it is very difficult to know if what they are doing is correct. Ideally, you would want to start with the more experienced person on the B side, paired with a beginner or less experienced person on the A side.

It should be mentioned that people often remark that the role of Player B (the receiver/sendee) is easier. It is easier to sense when you are being effectively "pushed" with the energy. For Player A, even if connected to Player B, the sensations of "sending" the energy are less noticeable at first. Player A will feel like they have "not done anything" even though Player B will be saying otherwise. So, Player A needs lots of practice to develop confidence in what they are doing. Player B should help Player A by "leading" them to their center and by telling Player A when they are or are not "on it".

Also, the more relaxed Player A can be and the more chi that Player A has gathered in the lower dan tien the more success Player A will have. Be patient. Be supportive of one another. Practice.

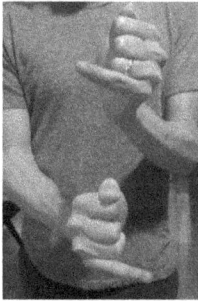

Player A Extends Fingers   *Player B Squeezes Fingers*
The joined hands are lined up on the centerline, spine to spine.

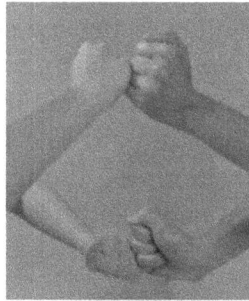

Once the Search has been done successfully several times while using the direct "spine to spine" alignment of the hands, Player A can move Player B's arms to various other positions and try to "Search Center" from the new configuration. Similarly, Player A can let Player B move the arms to a new position, and then Player A will have to "Search Center" from that location.

There are many variations to how this exercise can be done. Give it a try.

◆ ◆ ◆

The Horizontal "Search Center" Variation

A few of Master Wang's students who teach classes report that some of their students are more successful in their early "Search Center" interactions if they use this variation.

In this exercise Player A's role is again "active" in that he or she will be doing the "searching" to find Player B's center. Once the center is found, Player A will use the "internal energy", without physical force, to move Player B. The footwork and weight distribution remain the same, both parties are in the Archer's Stance with their left foot forward.

In this variation, Player A starts by making a fist with each hand. The hand is held vertically, the thumbs toward the ceiling and the back of the hands facing the side walls. Player A's arms are held about waist high with just a simple bend at the elbow joint. Then, Player A opens and extends the index and middle fingers of each hand together as a pair. The ring and little fingers remain in the closed fist position; the thumb of each hand folds in towards the palm, lightly touches and remains resting on the closed ring finger.

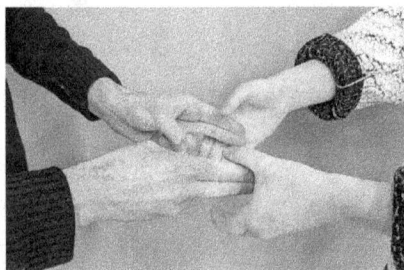

Player A extends the index and ring fingers.

Player B, with his or her arms also bent at the elbows, then grasps and squeezes Player A's two extended fingers (index and middle) of each hand with a firm but not too tight grip. Both players should move their elbows outward a little so their combined arms are making a slightly rounded shape. The result is that the partners are now making a more or less circular shape between them which is about waist level high and parallel to the floor.

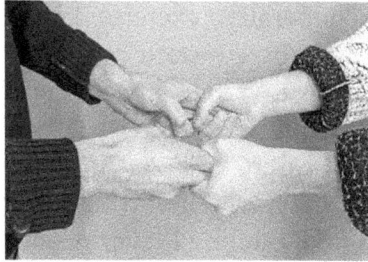

Player B squeezes the extended fingers firmly but not too tight.

Having done so, the partners are now connected physically but may not be connected energetically unless they have some experience doing "Search Center" already. To help Player A make the energetic connection, Player B will slightly extend his or her grip forward and put a quite small but noticeable amount of pressure/force in a forward direction toward Player A but without actively pushing forward with his or her arms. As in the first exercise, when the energetic connection is made both parties will be able to sense/feel it. Remember that both players need to start from their Center when making the energetic connection.

Just as before, Player B must maintain a gentle yet firm grip (not too tight) and Player A must continue to use his or her mind/intent (*Yi*) throughout the search until Player B's center and balance have been compromised to the extent that Player B moves. In conducting the horizontal search, Player A may find it useful to imagine that Player B's arms are like the ends of a turkey's wishbone which converge at Player B's spine. Player A just extends the chi along those lines until the energy converges on Player B's center point. It is important that Player A maintain the "Globe Shape" and not allow it to "collapse"; and yet, Player A cannot physically push back against Player B's slight pressure. The "Globe Shape" is maintained via Player A's relaxed (*Sung*) and rooted connection to the ground. Player A must use sensation and mind/intent (Yi) to extend the chi along the desired path. Player A should concentrate on the sensations associated with sending/extending the chi and not worry about having to move Player B. If Player A can find Player B's center and maintain the mental focus, Player B will certainly be moved as a result.

Again, this is a cooperative exercise. Player B should maintain the firm squeeze and slight, constant pressure throughout because that will enable Player A to better sense where Player B's Center is located. When first learning this exercise, Player B should not hide the Center or resist the Search. If Player A is having difficulty finding their partner's center, Player B should help Player A by "leading" them to their center and by telling Player A when they are or are not "on it".

Once the Search has been done successfully from the initial position several times, the parties can then move the arms to other positions, including the vertical spine to spine circular alignment used during the Pinkie Grab exercise. When doing so it is important to keep the circular shape/globe shape of the partners' paired arms intact. The parties can also change the weight distributions and which leg is forward in the Archer's Stance.

Another more advanced variation is to have Player B stand in front of a sturdy chair or bench during the exercise. Player A then uses the internal energy to compromise Player B's Center in a manner that makes Player B bend at the waist/hips and sit down on the chair or bench. Particularly at first, this requires good listening skills (*ting jin*) by both parties. The goal on both sides is to sense and understand the flow, direction, and amount of energy. This should be done carefully. This is not done by Player A using physical force *(Li)* to shove Player B backward or down!

After several searches, the partners then change roles so that Player B will be the one conducting a search and Player A will be the one responding to the search.

◆◆◆

Appendix C: The Seated Pull

A "Search Center" Exercise

One of the training exercises that Master Wang has his students perform is the "Seated Pull". It involves sitting on a chair or bench and seeing if your partner can disturb your seated position by pulling steadily on your outstretched arm.

The "sitter" positions his or her body on the front edge of the chair or bench with the sit bones near the edge. The upper body is held in the same relaxed manner as you would use at the start of the solo tai chi form. The torso is upright, the head is suspended from above, the chin tucked in slightly to allow the "Jade Pillow" gate at the base of the skull to open, the low back and the abdominal muscles are relaxed and free of unnecessary tension, the body is centered in the lower dan tien, the *kwa* (kua) and the leg muscles are relaxed, and the feet are flat on the ground about shoulder-width apart.

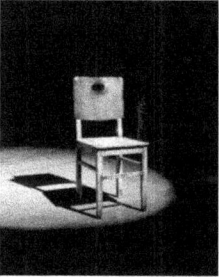

The sitter extends an arm and the "puller" grasps the outstretched palm like executing a handshake. Sometimes the puller will use two hands, one in the handshake grip and the other grasping the sitter's wrist. Once the two people are attached in this manner, the puller begins to apply a slow but steadily increasing amount of pull on the sitter's arm in an effort to disturb the sitter's posture and perhaps even pull him or her up and out of the seated position.

The sitter's task is to transfer that pulling force through the body and into the feet so that the force of the pull goes directly into the floor. This must be done without the sitter offering physical resistance in the form of strength or muscular tension in his or her own body. If the puller was to suddenly let go, the sitter who uses muscular resistance will react backward and lose his or her balance. So, the sitter seeks to keep the body aligned but relaxed. When done properly, the puller feels as if they were trying to lift the entire earth and the sitter does not move. This has little or nothing to do with the relative size or strength of the two people. When properly aligned and suitably connected a smaller seated person can readily neutralize a much stronger and larger one. It can be done with ease but it is not easy at first.

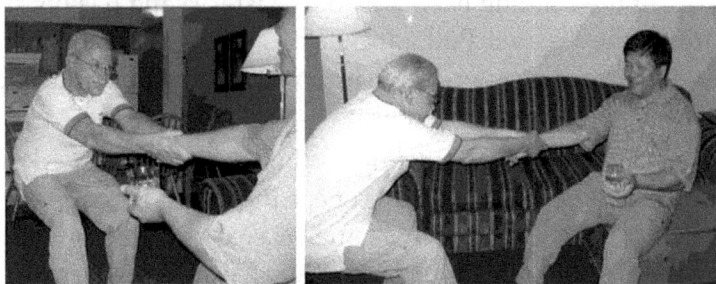

Master Wang Demonstrates Seated Pull Exercise

From the sitter's point of view, the task is both mental and physical. It must begin with the correct physical alignment throughout the body, particularly of the shoulder of the extended arm. "Coordination" is one of Master Wang's Seven Principles. (See Chapter 9.) This principle can have different meanings in different contexts. Here it involves the unification of the physical structure of the body in a way where all the skeletal parts are aligned and positioned so that the body itself has become one unified structure, like the ironwork frame of a building, and the Center is maintained.

One of the constant corrections any student of tai chi hears is to keep the shoulders down or let the shoulders relax, etc. One of the results of this lowering of the shoulders is that the shoulder blade itself becomes more securely attached to the back of the rib cage such that the two areas seem almost fused. They become integrally connected to the rest of the body yet without any tension or force being used to achieve this result. Relaxing the various muscle groups in the shoulder girdle and back allows the various parts to simply fit together in a more harmonious and integrated manner.

• *An Important Word of Caution:* The sitter is the person who controls the exercise. They say when the puller should start or stop the pulling motion. The puller should stop immediately if the sitter requests it. When trying this, if you do, please remember that the puller should pull slowly, gently, and only gradually increase the force and strength of the pull. This is a cooperative learning exercise, not a competition. The puller should never suddenly yank or jerk the partner's arm or use a sudden burst of brute force. You do not want to injure the shoulder of the sitter. The puller's goal is to assist the sitter in realizing when he or she has attained the correct alignment and integration of the body so that the puller now "feels" the floor. There is nothing to "win".

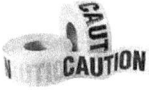

So, back to the chair sitting exercise. In the beginning, the puller is usually able to interfere with the sitter's composed posture quite easily. The sitter's first tendency is to resist the pull by offering a countervailing muscular effort, usually with the muscles of the arm and shoulder. The stronger person simply "wins" of course. The sitter then decides to not offer muscular resistance. He or she lets the extended arm slacken. This does not work either. The pulled arm is almost immediately extended to its full length, the elbow joint becomes locked and the arm becomes gently stretched away from its socket, the torso starts to rotate or come forward a little, the body bends at the waist and the puller "wins" again.

So, letting the pulled arm relax and fully extend in that manner was not the apparent solution either. The sitter should not let the pulled arm be fully extended. The better position for the pulled arm is to keep the elbow down like in the "Lift Hands" or "Play Guitar/Pipa" form postures. With practice, the sitter will find the best position.

The sitter must also recall the companion lesson from the form that the shoulders must be relaxed. One of the "tricks" for the sitter to learn is to make sure that the shoulder blade of the pulled arm is relaxed and attached to the back of the rib cage. A better position can be found if the sitter first rolls the shoulders up and forward and then reverses that action by rolling the shoulders up, back, and downward. If standing, the position of the slack arms would then be such that the middle fingers would be aligned with the side-seam that runs vertically down the outside of your pant leg. In this back and downward position, it is as if the shoulder blade becomes gently "wedded" or united with the rib cage. From this down and relaxed position, the pulled arm is not pulled out of the joint. Instead, the force pulling on the arm is more readily able to be transferred down through the body and into the sitter's feet and the floor beneath.

"Concentration" is another of Master Wang's Seven Principles. (See Chapter 9.) For the sitter, maintaining one's Concentration in the lower dan tien and "ignoring" the puller's efforts to unseat them is another essential component of this exercise. Of course, the sitter will feel the pull but can choose not to be unduly concerned about it. Instead, the sitter should maintain focus on the lower dan tien and concentrate his or her mind exclusively on the idea of "down" or "sinking their Center (lower dan tien) into the floor and ground.

When properly aligned and unwaveringly mentally focused it takes very little effort or strength to be able to respond appropriately to the force of the slow, steady pull. The puller seems to be, and is, working rather hard while the sitter can remain relaxed and untroubled. With repetitive, cooperative practice this response to being pulled becomes automatic and is a revelation to all concerned. (See Appendix E, Use the Mind, Not Force.)

Practice slowly and carefully. Remember that the sitter controls the starting and stopping. Give helpful verbal feedback. Be patient with one another.

A Standing Position Variation

This "Search Center" exercise can also be done from a standing position. This is a more advanced variation in which the person being tested adopts an Archer's Stance with the body centered and the weight distributed 50/50 in the manner advocated by Master Wang. It requires even more coordination and integration of the entire body, upper and lower, and expanded concentration as well. When done properly, the puller will feel like they are pulling the weight of the earth while their partner simply remains centered and relaxed.

This standing variation is best attempted after students have been repeatedly successful in the Seated Pull exercise. In the standing position, it is a common mistake for students to lean backward and revert to the use of physical strength *(Li)* to resist the increasing force of the constant, gentle pull. This is readily seen if the puller suddenly relaxes or releases his or her grip. A person using *Li* or leaning backward will often move backward and even lose their balance. Such mistakes can be better avoided by first mastering the Seated Pull. Training in this manner takes time and patient practice.

◆ ◆ ◆

Appendix D: Recollections & Reflections
from
Senior Students

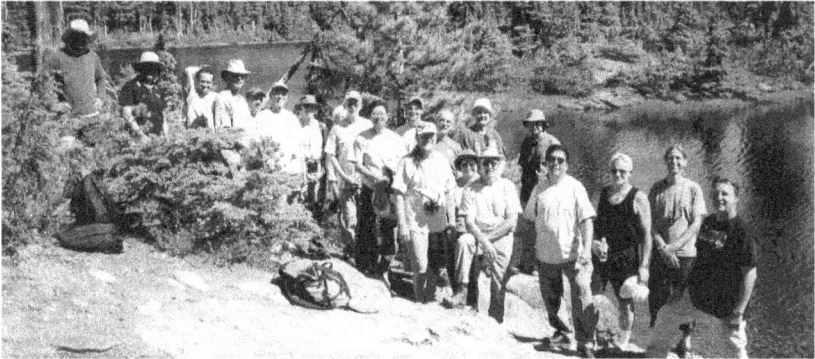

The following pages contain recollections and reflections gathered from various senior students concerning their experiences with Master Wang and the lessons learned.

♦ ♦ ♦

My Teacher, My Friend

I started my tai chi journey in 1970, half a century ago. At the time I thought it would be a fun, "cool" exercise to learn. Never did I imagine it would become a life-long path of personal growth and health, both physical and spiritual. My current dedication to tai chi form practice and "Search Center" partner work is because of Master Henry Wang.

Meeting Master Wang in 1983 changed my life for the better; and, outside of my parents and immediate family, he has been the major mentor for me.

He has taught me tai chi philosophy, form, and partner practice. That could have been enough, but more importantly, he has been an example to me of commitment and love for an ancient Chinese discipline that has applications to my life. Tai chi is his life, and it is rare to encounter someone so focused and dedicated to a particular field of study. No day goes by where he isn't studying tai chi and striving to improve and disseminate his knowledge. He is an example to me of what is possible.

In addition to instilling a love for tai chi, and teaching me that I can always do better, he has influenced my life in many other ways. He loves me and my family and his students. As a master, he feels responsible for our lives. He contacts us frequently to see how we are doing. He listens and offers advice to us when there are issues in our lives. He demands excellence from us but accepts us when we don't meet his expectations. He is not perfect, of course, but he consistently "walks the walk". He is always positive, even when others would be discouraged. He has great talents but doesn't try to prove himself to others.

Were it not for Master Wang, I probably would have given up tai chi long ago. He showed how the practice is more than an exercise. I need to challenge myself daily both physically and mentally. My health has benefited. I have contacts around the world who share our Master and who have added to my life. My professional work has been influenced beneficially and I am more at ease with my family and friends.

Master Wang is my tai chi master and a true and loyal friend.

Peter Uhlmann, M.D.

Powell River, B.C.

大徒弟

dà tú dì

(Longstanding/oldest apprentice/disciple)

How I Met Master Henry Wang

In 1986 I heard from my chiropractor that a Tai Chi master had moved from Taiwan to Powell River on the British Columbia mainland, a reasonably short ferry ride across the Georgia Strait from my home near Courtenay on Vancouver Island.

I had been learning and practicing Tai Chi since 1984 and had found a teacher, Judith Weaver, who had studied with Master Cheng Man-ch'ing. I had seen films of Master Cheng's form and read some of his writings and I trusted in the lineage quite completely. Judith was a strong teacher and I felt I was in the best possible hands.

I was very dismissive of the story of a "Master" being in Powell River. I surmised that everyone from Taiwan who did Tai Chi considered themselves to be a "Master". I already had a direct connection to the teachings of Master Cheng and was in no mood to try a new teacher.

My chiropractor gave me a Powell River phone number and I told him I'd call.

The next part of the story is that at the time I had been taking some personal development courses. One of the precepts was to consider your word to be your life. Even though I had NO desire to call the number, I carried it around for weeks knowing that I would call but wishing I hadn't said I would.

When I finally did call it was Peter Uhlmann's house but Henry Wang picked up the phone. After some talk, I asked him to come to Courtenay and give a demonstration to our tai chi group. I was able to get a meeting room in Courtenay and picked him up at the ferry from Powell River. A solid Chinese man walked up the ramp and I had no difficulty realizing it was Henry.

Ten or twelve of us watched that day as he did his form for us. By this time, I had seen many different people do Tai Chi and I was shocked at how different the quality of his movement was from anything I had witnessed before. It was as if a cyclone was moving inside his body with the outside slowly and powerfully following the inside current.

I was so overwhelmed with the demonstration that I asked if I could set up some classes in Courtenay for him until he went back to Taiwan in the late fall. He agreed and getting people to sign-up for the classes seemed easy. After I had checked the students in, I would take a place at the rear of the room and follow along with every class. I was privileged to have so many classes and realized that at the level at which he taught, I needed all the repetition I could get.

Master Wang (as I now realized he was) immigrated to Canada in late 1987 with his wife Ivy and their children David and Amy. Peter Uhlmann and I met them at the Vancouver Airport with a van for them and their luggage. Chinatown was the first stop and I can still remember little Amy reaching up to grasp my little finger as we stood on the street.

Regular classes in Courtenay soon followed and Henry usually stayed at my house.

Now it`s thirty-plus years on from then and I have never missed a day of Tai Chi practice.

To have found the WAY is a wonderful thing.

Lawrie Milne
Courtenay, B.C.

290

Some Things I've Learned

After 30 years of studying tai chi with Master Wang, I have been *thinking about what I have learned and acquired from being with him. I have learned that Centre is more than dan tien. Being centred is being at peace and in harmony with the world and those around me. I have come to realize that it is not mastery that is important but being grounded, relaxing, and letting go. One of his favourite expressions is "Invest in Loss". Give up that ego. The internal line we follow, the flowing, is, on another level, The Way, the path we follow in life. Everything is connected by that line. I have also come to see that the spiral is not revolving around the self. It grows ever larger and encompasses everyone and everything around us.*

Several years ago, Master Wang gave me a gift. It was a smooth, polished stone with the word "BALANCE" etched into it. It was a timely gift as I had been experiencing a great deal of turmoil in my life and it caused me to stop and reflect. Balance is more than standing on one foot. It is also a kind of internal equilibrium…balancing all the forces flowing through you and coming at you, your relationships and responsibilities, and your emotions.

I have learned that it is far beyond mastering the Tai Chi form. It is a philosophy, a map, of how to live your life fully. At the end of technique is skill, at the end of skill is transcendence.

Ann Z

Comox, B.C.

Going the Soft Way

My wife and I started tai chi almost 30 years ago knowing only that old people were doing it. It seemed to be a good way to maintain flexibility and balance as we aged. I knew nothing about it as a martial art and certainly knew nothing about Master Henry Wang.

I struggled while trying to learn the order of the form's postures but persisted. Along with learning form, we began to learn about Chinese culture and philosophy as well. The real draw was getting involved in authentic Chinese food. Visits to Master Wang's house always involved sipping tiny cups of horribly bitter tea. It took some time before we realized that if we didn't want more, we should leave the cup full. Eventually, we began to appreciate the subtleties of real tea and develop a love of fine tea. As our understanding of tai chi began to increase, we became more and more immersed in both the culture and our friendship with Master Wang and his wife, Ivy.

Master Wang introduced us to "Search Centre"; and, as I ventured out to meet with other tai chi players, I began to appreciate the beauty and effectiveness of "Search Centre" compared to traditional Push Hands practice. No one I met could come close to matching Master Wang's softness, nor his explosive power. Although everyone pays lip service to softness, no one truly can understand the degree to which it can be taken unless touched by Master Wang.

After more than 25 years we are part of an international group of players who share a passion for tai chi. We have dear friends from afar we see only once a year at our annual Mt Washington summer camp as well as a large local community of people who come from many different backgrounds, all held together by our common dedication to the art. Yes, we have maintained and even improved our balance and flexibility and gained so much more!

Joe Z

Comox, B.C.

292

Advancing the Art of Tai Chi

The first time I heard about Master Wang was in the late 1980s. At the time, he was teaching Tai Chi in Powell River and Comox, British Columbia. He was an old neighbor and my wife's friend from Taiwan. He would call her occasionally at our home in Toronto concerning questions he had about the Canadian immigration process.

I first met him in 1991. In November 1991, my two friends, James Wang (Master Wang's former student and "Search Center" partner in Taiwan) and William Chu (a Kendo Master and Summer Camp student) and I sponsored a one-week visit to Toronto for him. During that visit, I began to learn Master Wang's Tai Chi form and had my first "Search Center" experience.

I can still remember the following incident clearly in my mind. It was late afternoon in William's home, and I had an opportunity to do "Search Center" with Master Wang. As instructed, I reached out and made contact to start "One Hand Circling". Suddenly, my body began to fly and my back hit the wall with a loud thud. However, I quickly realized that my body still functioned properly and did not feel any pain at all. Furthermore, the wall was not damaged. I was amazed by this action and started to appreciate the softness and power of Chi. While I had learned different forms of Tai Chi before, this experience motivated me to begin transforming from my old form to Master Wang's Tai Chi form.

Before I met Master Wang in person, I had already been a Tai Chi student for a few years. I had learned the simplified 24 posture form, the 48 posture form, the 108 posture Yang Style form, the Chan Style form, and a Tai Chi sword form as well. It had taken me about five years to learn these various Tai Chi forms which is why I struggled quite a bit before I gave them up to learn Master Wang's Tai Chi form.

In the summer of 1992, my family decided to take a trip from Toronto to visit Master Wang and his family in Comox, B.C. We were kindly invited to stay at their home. Each day my wife and I followed him in *doing morning exercises at nearby forest parks. However, while changing to his form, I was still holding onto my old Tai Chi forms and practiced them myself in addition to what Master Wang was teaching me.*

The following year, in June of 1993, Master Wang's wife Ivy visited us from Comox along with her mother and daughter. As I was having difficulties trying to learn his form, Ivy graciously helped me learn the first section of it.

By 2007, my transformation from my old Tai Chi routine to this new Tai Chi routine had been completed. This was certainly a milestone for my journey in learning Tai Chi. First of all, I managed to finish learning all three sections of the Tai Chi form on both sides of the body. Secondly, I was able to practice his Tai Chi form free from the influence of the other forms I had previously studied. By this milestone, I had completely established a new daily routine for myself and was feeling good.

The first summer camp I attended was in July 1999 and I have been attending the camps regularly ever since. Throughout the years Master Wang has promoted the philosophy of Lao Tzu in connection with his instructions on how to correctly practice Tai Chi form and "Search Center". Among other things, Master Wang advocates that you should practice the Tai Chi form with the idea that it has no shape and no martial arts purpose. Practicing with this mindset will improve the circulation of Chi.

Whenever I watched Master Wang demonstrate the Tai Chi form, I saw that he managed to make each of the moves so softly, so gently, and so smoothly. It made me think that this was the way we were supposed to practice the form. In learning from him what good quality form looks like I admire his achievements a lot more.

Master Wang has devoted his life to the study and teaching of Tai Chi. In doing so he has accomplished several important advancements in the art. He has developed his Seven Principles for Tai Chi Practice which apply to all styles of Tai Chi. He has revised the traditional Tai Chi forms, such as Cheng Man-ch'ing's style, and developed them into Wang's Tai Chi form. He has advocated for important changes to the rules of competitive Tai Chi and promoted "Search Center" to replace Push Hands. These contributions to the Tai Chi movement are significant. This is why I believe sooner or later, what he did will be recorded in the great history of Tai Chi development.

Tak J. Kong
Toronto, Ontario

From Rugby to Tai Chi

There have been two recreational passions in my life, rugby and tai chi. During the summer of 1987, I seriously injured my back and discovered that I was unable to continue my usual daily fitness routine of jogging a few miles. Fortunately for me, Shifu had recently started teaching tai chi at the Courtenay Recreation Center on northern Vancouver Island. Having ignored any remedial recreation for my broken body for as long as possible, I was now ready to participate in a new activity. One which I hoped that I could share with others in the same way I had shared my love of rugby. So, shortly after I turned forty-five, I joined his tai chi class and that was my introduction to Master Henry Wang, my Shifu.

Push Hands vs. "Search Center": For thirty years, as both a rugby player and coach, I thrived on aggressive body contact but my injuries had limited my rugby-playing days. Push Hands, one of tai chi's competitive skills involving a test of balance between two contestants, was an ideal substitute activity to satisfy my need for physical contact. Each Sunday many of Shifu's students would meet outside at Comox Elementary School to practice Push Hands. I looked forward to each Sunday session. Initially, senior students complained that I was physically hard and too aggressive. Softness was alien to me. How could anyone push without applying physical force?

Master Wang, himself a Push Hands champion, had gone on to develop a new approach for such "competitive" tai chi encounters. He called it "Search Center". He often scolded us, "No, you're being too physical. "Search Center" should never result in a hard push!" We felt obliged to comply with his instruction, but in the heat of the moment soon lost interest in trying to understand his directions and returned to our more physically forceful and aggressive Push Hands habits. Now, after more than twenty-five years of form practice and "Search Center" encounters, I am honoured to be complimented on my 'softness', especially when it's offered by Shifu.

296

From "Search Center" to "No Touch": Over the years, Shifu has continuously refined his "Search Center" practices. He has emphasized to us that we need to use our mind (our Yi) and not physical force (our Li) while doing our form and in "Search Center" partner work. In improving his skills, he has investigated and developed a new level of refinement which he calls "No Touch".

Eventually, I became one of Shifu's students who responded to "No Touch". I recall the first moment vividly. We were at Lake Helen Mackenzie during one of the early summer camps. From about fifteen feet away, Shifu tried to move me using only his chi. I stood motionless waiting for something to happen. Anything! I had no idea what to expect. After what seemed like minutes, I decided to move and he seemed relieved. I had faked the response because I didn't feel any of the sensations that I usually felt when I physically approached and made contact with him.

Later, I realized that I had not connected to his Center as I usually did when I approached to engage him during a demonstration. The next time he tried "No Touch", I visualized connecting to his Center as I would if I was about to make physical contact. Sure enough, I was moved by his chi. The stronger I made the visualized connection, the stronger and more abruptly his chi affected me. If I visualized making a rugby tackle on him, he easily bowled me over even when I was ten feet or more from where he stood. This fits with the concept that tai chi is a remarkable martial art or an art of self-defense. Check out this picture of Shifu and me from his website. It shows what happens.

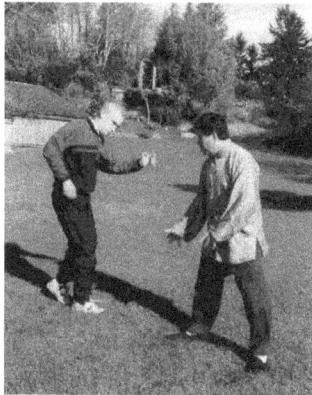

I believe that when I approach Shifu, my energy field extends in an attempt to connect with his Center. Shifu can sense my energy boundary and my body's Center. His clear awareness enables him to easily move me by directing a laser-like beam of chi at my Center. In response, my body behaves like a wind-blown tumbleweed broken free of its mooring.

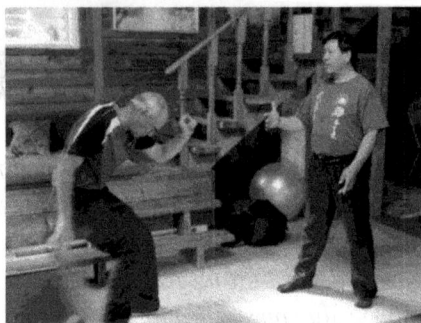

A Fortunate Invitation: *Over thirty-five years ago Peter and Ronnie Uhlmann spent some time in Taipei studying Chinese culture and language. When they asked for a good tai chi master, they were told that Henry Wang was one of the best teachers of Cheng Man-ch'ing's Yang Form in Taipei. Fortunately for all of us, Ronnie asked Shifu if he was interested in coming to Canada to teach tai chi.*

I am grateful to have had the privilege of studying with such a gifted and generous tai chi Master. After years of questioning and practicing, I have a true appreciation of what Shifu has offered us. His dedication to the perfection of his form and his astonishing "soft power" constantly surprises and inspires me. I am also thankful for the many tai chi friends and experiences that I have gained as a result of this ongoing study. The tai chi mystery will continue to be a challenge for us to collectively solve.

I am honoured to have been asked to write about some of my experiences with Master Wang. Thank you, Shifu.

James Milne
Comox, B.C.

298

A Personal Account of Tai Chi's Practice Benefits

Tai chi is a major focus in my life. I have received many benefits from my study of this ancient art form. Above all, I have learned to focus my attention internally instead of outwardly or "out worldly", and this has made a huge difference in both my practice and my overall well-being.

My internal focus started with noticing the positioning of my hands, arms, legs, feet, centre axis, and dan tien while doing the form. Then came more awareness of internal movement and a feeling of internal energy that I could sense inside my body. Energy that sometimes felt like a vibration, tingling, heat, or a sense of embodied aliveness.

Recognition of that internal presence of movement and space has provided relaxation and quieted the babbling mind. I now sense subtlety, flow, openness, and relaxation. My stress level is reduced; my physical and psychological body is more at ease. Of late, I am realizing that tai chi is a continuous path of learning, self-realization, awareness, spaciousness, and relaxation. One does not arrive at a final achievement; one experiences and becomes one with the experience.

Another aspect of tai chi is the development of community. Practicing form together as a group connects me to the larger group and engaging in "Search Centre" connects me to individuals. When engaged in "Search Centre" with another person I not only feel my internal energy I also sense the other person's internal energy. So, I am internally connected to self and my partner. When I focus my attention on this internal, life force energy connection between us, it intensifies the internal connection.

Engaging in "Search Centre" and the form has enhanced my relationships both within and outside of tai chi. I am more at ease in relationships, more aware of relaxing into my internal (life force aliveness) energy, and better connected to my root (releasing and receiving energy through my feet from the ground) which allows ease, relaxation, and clarity.

During my many years of studying with Master Wang, I have realized how important it is to have good guidance. Sifu provides a living example of the tai chi form that incorporates all his Seven Principles and witnessing this has greatly enhanced my practice. I also take weekly classes from Master Wang's wife, Ivy, and I have benefited from her diligence and attention to detail in practicing the form.

Working together with other students to practice, assess, and discuss what we are learning is all part of the process which has strengthened my practice. And of course, my overall health has progressed as well as my comfort level with relationships and life.

Practicing tai chi daily is important to maintain one's level of progress and to increase one's internal awareness and skill level. I was in my early twenties when I first saw someone practicing tai chi. I did not know what it was then, and I thought. Why would anyone do "those strange" moves with their bodies? Well, now I know, and I don't find it "strange"; instead, I find it wonderful (filled with wonder). I am very grateful and appreciative to have received the opportunity to study and practice tai chi with Master Wang, with his wife Ivy, and with all my fellow students. Thank you to all.

Summer McGee
Courtenay, B.C.

Eat Bitter to Know Sweet

I remember the first time I heard this Taoist saying from my teacher and it was to stay with me ever since.

Back in the early days of our annual Tai Chi summer camp, we had developed into a great group of friends. The third week in July was beginning to be our yearly reunion at the scenic Mt. Washington ski resort. It was a time to catch up as well as studying Tai Chi.

At camp, our days begin early. Starting around 6:00 a.m., we usually do an outdoor session of Chi Kung and Tai Chi form practice for about an hour or so. Then we return to our rooms to get ready for breakfast and the rest of the day's practice. One year, about mid-week, we started our usual post-breakfast, late morning class. That session consists of about 1.5 hours of form correction practice and 1.5 hours of "Search Center" practice. We students were in a jovial mood and there was much merriment going on during this session.

Well, we could see an eventual change in Master Wang's demeanor, especially as it was getting close to the end of the class and almost lunchtime. Let me add that we are practicing every day for several hours and hiking several miles in the mountains during the afternoons, so we are looking forward to our meals when that time comes around. So, this particular day as lunchtime approached and we could see and smell the food as the resort staff brought out the lunch items, we certainly were ready for class to end and lunch to begin. But that was not to be.

Master Wang just kept us going with more form practice and more "Search Center". Eventually, we could hear the resort staff taking back the lunch items as it was over two hours past the time we were supposed to have lunch. Finally, Master Wang ended the class and we were dismissed. Completely exhausted and very hungry we were more than a bit confused about what just transpired.

That evening at dinner time Master Wang asked us how the food tasted. Of course, we all said how amazing it tasted and that we were so

301

hungry. It was then he shared the idea of "to eat bitter to know sweet". He said that he felt that there was too much playing around during the early morning class and that showed disrespect for him and the art. He shared that only through diligent practice with a sincere heart can our level grow. It is through hard work and with some sacrifice will you eventually taste the "sweet" that the practice provides. That we needed to eat bitter to know the sweet of the art.

I also saw another lesson in this. Our teacher, after many years of hard and devoted practice, his period of eating bitter, was now willing to share the sweet, the fruits of his knowledge with us. That fact was something to appreciate, to respect, to admire, and be thankful for.

Paul Seronko
Bend, Oregon

Squeeze My Arm

I originally started studying tai chi in the late '70s when I met a woman who was teaching the long-form (108 posture) Yang Style. Like many people of my generation, I had seen and become intrigued with tai chi from the memorable scene in the 1969 movie "Easy Rider" and so I jumped at the chance to try it out. Unfortunately, after only a month or two of class, my teacher moved away. I enjoyed the practice so I kept at it on my own for a few months but then eventually let my practice lapse.

I had another chance at learning tai chi in the early '80s. My sister married and her husband began to teach me both Wu Style tai chi and Tae Kwon Do, the Korean martial art known for its formidable kicks. I found out the hard way, what Master Wang has said many times since, that it is not possible to study hard and soft martial arts simultaneously. So, before long, both fell by the wayside as well.

In 1996 I ruptured a disc and had back surgery. Sometime before that, I had met a tai chi teacher who unbeknownst to me was one of Master Wang's senior students. After my surgery, I began to study tai chi with him as rehabilitation for my back surgery. I have not had a significant issue with my back since resuming my tai chi practice. Even so, my tai chi might have lapsed once again had I not met Master Wang himself.

In 1998 he came to my hometown, Boise, Idaho to conduct a workshop. Even though it was a fairly basic workshop, I was impressed with Master Wang as a practitioner and as a person. I mentioned that I hoped I would be able to study with him more. He replied that it was up to karma. I continued attending classes after he left and practiced faithfully outside of class.

Master Wang returned to Boise in 2000 for another workshop. At that time, he was just starting to reveal his "No-Touch" skills to his students. I confess that I thought it bordered on magic. But, having experienced him doing it to me, I left that workshop even further motivated to continue my practice. I wanted to see if I too could learn to do it. In the years since I have become more interested in the health-related benefits of tai chi practice and for a while gave up on the idea of being able to do "no touch".

In July 2000, I also attended my first of Master Wang's annual tai chi summer camps. Since I knew no one in Canada, my teacher arranged for myself and my friends, Tom and Mark, to stay at Master Wang's house the day before camp. Of course, this meant rising early and going to the local park to practice.

After qigong and form practice, we each did some "Search Center" with him. At that time, it consisted of Master Wang having us stand in front of a park bench. Then he would direct us to grab his forearm tightly with both hands. When we did, he caused us to involuntarily sit down with seemingly no effort on his part. Our firm grip gave him information that enabled him to capture our center, but it seemed to me that there was something more going on. When I grabbed his arm, he kept telling me to squeeze harder but, try as I might, it felt to me as if I was barely touching him. It reminded me of trying to run in a dream where no amount of effort can make your legs move. It felt like somehow he was taking control of my muscles such that no matter how hard I tried, I couldn't clamp down on his arm.

Since then, I have attended almost all of his summer camps and have become a firm believer in the power of the mind and qi. I can even do some "No-Touch", in a very controlled situation with a sensitive partner.

I will likely never reach Master Wang's level, partly because of his natural talent, but mostly because I don't practice as much as he has and still does. He has been practicing 4-6 hours a day for 45 years while I have been practicing 30-90 minutes a day for 20 years. It's easy to see that it would be hard to catch up. However, one thing I have learned is that his ideas and principles work. Anyone willing to practice in accord with his principles and to put in the time required should be able to reach a high level.

Greg Harley
Boise, Idaho

The Five Elements Stone

I had only been studying taiji with Master Wang for a few years when I had the opportunity to take two weeks of private lessons with him at his home in Comox, British Columbia. At that point, I was still very early in my training and had more ambition than skill or sense. In retrospect, the majority of the significant lessons he taught me during that trip had more to do with understanding his taiji "lifestyle" and philosophy rather than just the minute details of the form or "Search Center". His first instruction to me when he picked me up from the airport was, "Watch how I live."

While some may think that taiji only happens during those moments when you practice the form or engage in Push Hands or practice taiji's martial applications, Master Wang's approach to the art is decidedly different. He lives taiji. Thus, any activity he engages in as he flows through his day is an opportunity for practicing his taiji.

One such activity happens to be searching for unique stones on the rocky Vancouver Island beaches that border Comox. We headed out on several such expeditions during my visit. Mind you, the stones which attract his interest are not the "pick up and put in your pocket" variety but are more along the lines of the dutiful student will "lug a 100-pound object up 200 steps from the beach" kind. Of course, the obvious taiji lesson for me on that particular outing was how to find the center of the day's chosen rock and how to use my center to carry it up the far too many steps back to the car. Which is just what I did. A heavy lesson learned I thought as I dumped it into the car. The more subtle and profound lesson came later once the rock reached its home in Master Wang's back yard.

He named that rock the "five elements stone" because it contained all the elemental colors in Chinese medicine (red, yellow, green, white, and black). Because the stone had been plucked from the briny waters of the Strait of Georgia (between mainland British Columbia and Vancouver Island), it was covered in small barnacles and seaweed. My task was to clean the rock up and reveal its underlying magnificence. So, being eager to please the Master, I began furiously scrubbing the stone and meticulously scraping every crevice. After ten minutes of this frenzied effort, Master Wang came over. Expecting appreciation for my efforts, much to my surprise, he instead told me that I was doing the assigned chore completely wrong. He said, "Cleaning the stone is like taiji practice. Don't focus on the small details! It takes many years of rubbing the rock to make it shiny. You can't see the progress in just one day. Taiji is like this. Just practice a little every day, that's all. Eventually, you will see the result."

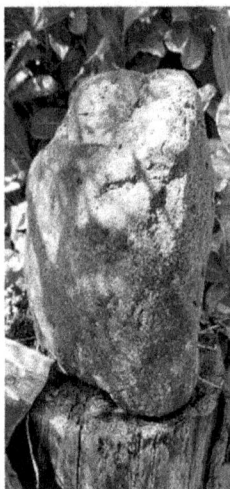

The Five Elements Stone

Now, several years later, I realize more and more that was the true lesson of the day. It's easy to get bogged down and burned out trying to create perfection with the taiji form and its applications. This can paralyze both the beginner and a long-time student as there are so many elements of taiji (physical, mental, and philosophical) that can be focused on. Master Wang's simple instruction to simply practice, helped sustain my taiji studies when I was conflicted with ideas of obsessive perfection or if I was worried that my taiji wasn't as "good" as someone else's. The five elements stone still lives in Master Wang's back yard and I'm reminded of this wisdom each time I visit his home. And while I don't have a five elements stone to polish, I do have the "Seven Principles" in the taiji form that

306

require daily attention. My job is to show up daily and do the work. "Just practice a little every day, that is all!"

Chris Bryhan

Bend, Oregon

http://www.westpinetaichi.com

On Meeting Master Wang

Since I was a teenager, I have been searching for, training, and studying martial arts. Many different styles have interested me, and although I only studied a few, the styles that I did train, seemed to come into my life when I was ready for a change or needed to grow in different ways. Tai chi entered my life, in exactly this way.

I started at age twelve with one year of karate. Then I spent the next five years, on and off, learning Taekwondo, the Korean art known for its various kicks. (Master Wang also studied it while in the ROC army. So, we have that in common.) It was then around age twenty that I discovered Thai kickboxing. This was it I thought. From the first time that I saw the Thai fighters kicking, elbowing, and kneeing the pads and bags with such relaxed power, I knew that this was a martial art I wanted to train. I soon became completely focused and devoted to Muay Thai. Unfortunately, a few years later a work injury and a Muay Thai sparring injury resulted in my giving up kickboxing permanently. I then began attending Iyengar Yoga classes to help heal my body.

I can recall during those years I was training Muay Thai, that I felt a calling on numerous occasions to explore tai chi. Some inner voice was telling me tai chi was the 'ultimate' martial art, and that I needed to study it. I knew little about it. With no internet or YouTube to help my research, I started reading books and going to watch various classes to learn more about this mysterious art. It was a series of serendipitous events, that I now see as blessings in my life, that led me away from the hardstyle path I was on and headed me toward the soft way of tai chi.

In 2002, at age 28, I left my native Australia to travel the world for two years. Along the way, I learned a little tai chi in Granada, Spain, and some more from a Korean teacher on the north shore of Oahu, Hawaii. These first meetings during my travels opened my eyes to what tai chi might be about, and I was now inspired to find a good teacher or school and to dedicate myself to learning tai chi.

Whether coincidence or karma, around mid-May, 2005, I was traveling again and I decided to make a stopover in Baja Mexico. While there, I met a San Diego, California man who was a tai chi practitioner and enthusiast. He had competed in various tai chi Push Hands competitions and even won a few. We discussed tai chi often. He mentioned reading in magazines about this tai chi master, Henry Wang, who lived in British Columbia. My friend said that Wang knew of a lost secret Yang style form which had helped Wang develop his incredible chi powers. I was very interested in this news and thought it was a favorable sign in my own life. As I was already on my way to Canada, I decided I would go find Master Wang and see if I could study with him.

The day I met Master Wang for the first time, I walked into the Comox recreation center and he was sitting there talking with some of his students. This was in the fall of 2005 and I was thirty-one years old. As I entered, I recall him looking at me curiously. I introduced myself and told him that I had come from Australia and wanted to learn Tai chi. His first words were, "I think this is my good karma you have come here from so far to take my classes. I think one day you will go teach my tai chi in Australia. This is very good.". I was unsure how to take what he had just said, but was grateful and intrigued to be meeting a Master and able to take his classes in the quiet little town of Comox, British Columbia.

When I told Master Wang of my previous martial arts experience and the limited amount of tai chi training, he asked to see my tai chi form. I started demonstrating the first third of the Yang form I had learned. I had only performed a few postures when he stopped me. "Okay, that's enough. Thank you.", he said. I was surprised. I told him I hadn't finished and had more to show. He replied, "No need. It's empty form." What was "empty form"? I didn't understand what he meant. I had been practicing martial arts for nearly twenty years by then. My legs were strong, I felt like I had built up roots by getting down low in my stances, as I had been shown by the Yang style teachers. What was "empty"? Now, after nearly fifteen years of additional practice, I am happy to say that I am fortunate to begin to understand what he was referring to.

I recall thinking that much of the time the classes were a test. That I, and the other Westerners wanting to learn, were being tested to see if we were worthy or had what was needed to learn tai chi from a Master. I had read about the traditional Masters doing such things but had never experienced it before. Nor had I ever been taught by a Master for that matter.

During class, he would forget my name, or sometimes ignore me. Again, I would think, he is testing me to see how I react or if I would be offended and leave. I let these things go as I was determined to learn tai chi and felt blessed that I had been guided to study with a genuine master, albeit a challenging one at times. After a few weeks, I noticed he remembered my name and seemed friendlier towards me. It felt as if I had passed some early test of dedication or perseverance to be able to learn tai chi from him.

This was not the case for many in the class. The large group of beginners gradually diminished over the weeks. The training did not suit many Westerners' concepts of what tai chi is and it revealed their lack of understanding about just how difficult it is to learn and perform correctly. I relate the drop-out process to pulling weeds from the garden so the remaining flowers have more space and energy to grow stronger. Although perhaps difficult for the students to understand why such testing was needed, I believe he was testing the class to see who is going to be a serious and dedicated student and who is not. Once the term finished, and the cold weather began to arrive, I headed south to Mexico in my beat-up old car, to find somewhere warm to practice what I had learned.

In time I found myself in the small fishing/surf town of La Ticla in Michuocan. I spent two months there surfing, playing guitar, and practicing the seven postures of Master Wang's form that I had learned. I focusing on his Seven Principles and 50/50, 100/0 weight distribution concept. I remember having to 'unlearn' the previous Yang form I had been studying, and its traditional 70/30 weighting. Fortunately, I had not studied that form long enough for too many bad habits to be ingrained in my body.

Eventually, I returned to Australia, and subsequently got a new job, met a woman, got married and we started a family. Since our first meeting in 2005, I have returned to Canada as often as I can to attend Master Wang's summer camp, see my tai chi friends, and continue my studies. I practice daily and, as Master Wang had predicted when we first met, I teach a few students his tai chi. Each day, I strive to follow his example and adhere to the principles of his "tai chi lifestyle" in my own life.

Dennis Peska

Mullumbimby,
New South Wales,
Australia

♦ ♦ ♦

Appendix E: Training with Master Wang

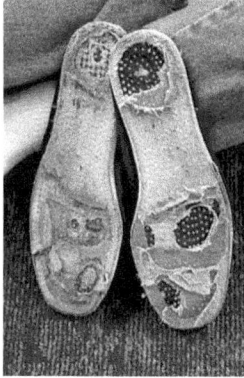

In the following pages the co-author, Ted Libby, describes several of his experiences while training with Master Wang.

♦ ♦ ♦

313

My First Encounter

(Chapter 6: Eastern Teacher, Western Students)

I first met Master Wang at a one-day workshop in Vancouver, British Columbia in November 1997. At that point, I had been studying Professor Cheng Man-ch'ing's tai chi style for five years in Seattle. As it turned out, Master Wang had also studied the same style at the Professor's Shr Jung School in Taipei, Taiwan. So, we at least had that much in common when I met him.

In those years, I was attending a two-hour class at least two and usually three times a week, including regular Push Hands and sword form practice in each class. I studied with various teachers but primarily with Saul Krotki and his Bear Palm Tai Chi Association group. In addition to his skills in Judo and other martial arts, Saul had been a direct student of Cheng Man-ch'ing for several years in New York City until the Professor died in 1975. To this day Saul's classes are devoted to preserving the tai chi principles and lessons he learned during his time with the Professor.

In my mind, I considered myself to be at least an "advanced beginner" when a number of us, including Saul, decided to attend Master Wang's workshop. Although that self-description was perhaps marginally accurate, I'm amused now when I think about how little I knew about tai chi then. The difference between what I thought I knew then and what I have since been exposed to and aspire to is so much more than I could've imagined. I was quite clueless really and operating quite contentedly in the world of the "unknown unknowns".

By the end of the day, that workshop had changed the ideas we all had about the potentials of tai chi. Personally, it also started me on an entirely different path in my tai chi life.

The *"Ward Off" Exercise:* Several interesting things happened to each of us that Saturday. However, for me, the single most astonishing aspect of the day occurred during a particular two-person exercise we were doing. Essentially the drill was a combination of posture testing and the

315

use of "fa jin" energy to toss your partner away. "Fa jin" means to issue or discharge power explosively from any particular tai chi posture. More often than not it is done incorrectly and entails excessive use of muscular force (Li).

The Set-Up for the Exercise: The exercise was cooperative, partner work training not "freestyle" Push Hands play. We would start with the "receiver/pushee" standing in an Archer's Stance (Bow Stance) with an arm extended in the "Ward-Off" (Peng) position. On the opposite side, the "sender/pusher "would stand in close in a similar stance. Once the pair was positioned, the sender/pusher would then just gradually and steadily increase the pressure of his "push" (An) on the "Ward Off" arm. The receiver/pushee's task was to both "absorb" the slowly increasing pressure and then demonstrate "fa jin" at some moment to repel the sender/pusher. After three or so tries on one arm, we would switch the "Ward-Off" to the leg and lead arm on the other side of the body. After three tries on that other side, we would then switch who did what.

What Just Happened? Everyone was engaged in this drill and we periodically switched from partner to partner around the room. When in the role of "receiver/pushee", I was having a terrible time with each person. My partner at the time was Mike, a friend and fellow student from Seattle who had been practicing tai chi for several years as well. Mike was having more success in both roles than I was. He and I had been alternating roles for a little while when Master Wang came over to observe.

As it happened, Mike was then taking the role of sender/pusher and I was his receiver/pushee. Naturally, both Mike and I stepped up the intensity of our interaction to demonstrate our respective "skills". If you've been in a similar situation, it should not surprise you to learn that in doing so we had markedly increased our use of strength and "dull force". Our efforts to make a good impression fell flat. Master Wang was certainly not impressed and rightfully so. Although I'm sure he had several helpful things to say to both of us, what I recall most clearly is what he did.

As receiver/pushee, I was standing with my right foot forward and my right arm in the "Ward-Off" position. Remember, my task in that role *was to use the "internal energy" but no physical force to bear up to Mike's incoming push and then to repel him using a type of "fa-jin".*

At this point in the story, I should admit that I didn't know very much about what "internal energy" entailed, what it felt like, or even how to cultivate it, let alone use it. I had read the literature and knew the theory well enough. However, I didn't know "the truth" of its feeling or function, either in solo form practice or in partner practice. Some things you just can't learn from books.

Master Wang stood behind me and slightly to the side. He had Mike start to push on my right arm a couple more times while he just watched. As eager as I was to do well, I was still unable to find the correct skeletal alignment and Mike easily overcame my muscular resistance. Then, perhaps after my third attempt, Master Wang placed the palm of his hand on my back at about the level of my right shoulder blade. In doing so, he said that neither one of us was using internal energy in our efforts. He then asked Mike to push again.

As Mike began his pushing action Master Wang applied just a slight amount of pressure but not force to my shoulder blade. Without any effort whatsoever on my part, Mike immediately crumpled and bent forward at his waist. His balance was completely compromised. As he doubled over, he was simultaneously propelled several steps backward. At the moment he'd pushed on my arm, it was as if Mike had just reached the end of a bungee-cord leap off a high bridge and was now in the initial rebound back towards the jump-off point. As a flailing Mike flew backward, I felt nothing, only a slight pulse, and a little penetrating warmth at the point of Master Wang's touch. Mike later said he too had felt nothing and just suddenly found himself hurtling backward at a rather alarming rate.

All wide-eyed and smiling as he walked back to us, Mike's immediate response was, "Do that again!" Master Wang just laughed, made a comment about using internal power, and simply walked on to the next pair. That was my startling introduction into the realm of "internal energy" and its potential power.

Despite having done a fair amount of Push Hands, I'd never seen or experienced anything like it and neither had Mike. I had done nothing. I'd only held up my arm. Mike was certainly "attached" to it at one moment but at the next, he wasn't. As Mike's push began, I hadn't moved my arm or body to "fa jin" and throw him back. Yet he'd been flung away. Neither one of us understood what happened.

That stunning and perplexing experience and the other events of that day changed my tai chi life completely. Mike and I had participated in a demonstration of the tai chi saying "four ounces can move a thousand pounds". There had been no fuss, no wasted movement, no struggle, no use of physical force. And even more amazingly, Master Wang had done this using my body and my arm as a conduit for the projection of his own "internal energy" into a second person. This was the "real deal" as far as I was concerned.

During the long drive back to Seattle, the entire conversation among the four of us in the car was about the inexplicable events of the day. The others all had their own unique and somewhat unsettling experiences with Master Wang's use of "internal energy" and we were eager to compare notes and theories.

The following Spring a few of us returned to Vancouver to attend another of Master Wang's workshops where similar events occurred. We again left mystified but satisfied and with the realization that tai chi was a much deeper study than we had previously imagined.

At those workshops, Master Wang spoke openly and at considerable length about "chi" and its cultivation during tai chi form practice. This was something I witnessed him use to great effect and I was keen to learn more about it from him. However, it wasn't until July 1999 that I had my next opportunity to study with Master Wang. That year I attended my first summer camp. He holds it each year during the third week of July at the Mt. Washington Alpine Resort outside of Comox, B.C. I've gone nearly every year since then and it is always a highlight of my summer.

Ted

The Pupil Stands Alone
(Chapter 7: Nurturing Fitness & Health)

It was winter. The temperature in Vancouver was in the low 30's and there was a remnant of light snow in the dormant flower beds scattered around Master Wang's front yard.

Their comfortable, two-story house was situated in a pleasant Vancouver neighborhood. In the springtime, cherry blossoms lined both sides of the road on this and surrounding streets. As was true for some other houses on the block, the bulk of the lot was below the grade of the sidewalk. Upon parking at the curb, you would cross the sidewalk and then descend four or five concrete steps to reach the walkway leading to the front porch.

Unless it was raining, which wasn't as frequent as you might imagine, we would practice tai chi in the front yard.

At that time, I had not been studying with Master Wang very long, maybe a year or less, maybe a little more. Overall, his instructions and training methods were contrary in many respects to what I had previously learned in the five years I'd been practicing tai chi before I met him. He quite simply contradicted all of my previous instructors on several major points.

The two most obvious differences were: (1) his insistence on turning the center/trunk before shifting the weight as opposed to shifting the weight and then turning the torso as I'd been originally taught, and (2) his directive not to bring the weight more than 50/50 into the front leg, which was certainly not the 70/30 split of weight in which I'd been so carefully schooled. Also, the timing of when the arms would move relative to the weight shift was quite different as well. New teacher, new approach to form practice. I was skeptical but willing.

That particular morning, after our customary two rounds of form, Master Wang gave me some specific instructions about a particular posture and the transition from it to the next. He demonstrated exactly what he wanted me to do in that short segment. Then, as he watched, I tried it a couple of times, incorrectly. Master Wang demonstrated again. I did my best once more but it was still not to his liking. I tried it yet again while he instructed me, step by step, as I did it. That time I got a little closer to what he had in mind. We worked on this little sequence together for a few minutes more.

"Okay, now practice.", he said and then promptly went inside the house.

There I was, alone in his front yard on this cold winter morning. Left to my own devices and with the simple directive to practice.

I resented it. After all, I'd driven over two hours from Seattle, and waited in line at the border to clear Canadian customs, and I was paying for this lesson, and it was freezing, and he wasn't there, and I didn't know what the hell I was doing really, and my hands were cold (you never wear gloves when you practice tai chi with Master Wang), and it was warm inside, and I wanted some tea. I resented all of it.

"Eat some bitter", I thought as I began my solitary practice. I'd read about things like this. How students were given little tests by their teachers. This must be such a test. Or, perhaps he just needed to use the restroom and would reappear momentarily.

Reluctantly, I practiced. Time passed. I got bored repeating the same short segment over and over and was no warmer for my efforts. Each hand was so cold that I was making a fist and blowing into it or rubbing the hands together to get the circulation moving. Where was the chi you might be wondering? So was I. In my defense, I might add this was early in my training with Master Wang. But, if the truth is told, it would be a few years later before my hands would occasionally warm up under such cold conditions.

Master Wang never did come back outside. I'm not sure how long I was out there on my own with my seething resentment and cold hands. It probably wasn't as long as it felt like but it was long enough for me to go through a whole range of reactions and emotions about the episode. Even so, I did practice the day's lesson.

Of course, in the final analysis, your practice must always be your own. Your teacher cannot practice for you. You are the one who must put in the time and do the work. That's the real "kung fu". That was certainly the most valuable part of that day's lesson.

At some point, Master Wang stepped out on the front porch and invited me back into the house. Leaving my resentment behind, I gladly stepped indoors. That morning's tea was some of the most welcome I'd ever had.

Ted

One Winter Morning
(Chapter 8: Development of Internal Chi)

My trips to Vancouver from Seattle frequently began with an unexpected call from Master Wang, usually in the middle of the week.

"I'll be in Vancouver this weekend, why don't you come up and visit?"

"Okay, I'll be there."

I'd often go up in the late afternoon on Friday and stay with him at their house.

On one Saturday morning, Master Wang and I got up early for the customary 6:00 A.M. practice in the front yard. This particular visit occurred in one of the early years of my trips to Vancouver. It was winter, January or February probably, and quite cold that morning, at least for Vancouver. The temperature was around freezing or perhaps a little less. What with Vancouver's latitude, the daylight might be barely visible but our day had begun.

Practice usually started with some chi kung exercises. There was no set number, pattern, or sequence that sifu would follow. Generally speaking, the exercises would work both the upper and lower body but I'd never know which particular exercise he would choose to include or exclude on any given morning. Mostly, I would just follow along as best I could. In the beginning, this involved a lot more looking over my shoulder than it did the actual practice of the drill. Eventually, I came to know most of the routine exercises and could cue off them almost simultaneously with his movement.

Following chi kung, Master Wang would lead at least two rounds of form. One performed from the usual right side and the other from the left. This two-sided practice is one of the first "breaks in tradition" that I encountered in his methods. The teachers in my tai chi lineage followed the Yang Style form as modified by Professor Cheng Man-ch'ing. I realize that many among those who practice the traditional Yang Family Style contend

322

that the Professor's style is not Yang Style at all. The whole topic of lineage, styles, and "correct" postures is better left for discussion another time, perhaps over a beer.

One of the things that attracted me to Master Wang as a teacher was his willingness to not only discuss the development of internal chi but also the heightened emphasis he puts on the student's task of striving for such development. Of course, everyone doing tai chi and many if not most of those who teach tai chi, talk, often at great length, about the wondrous and mysterious benefits of this chi. There is lots of such talk. However, in my then rather limited experience, I had not met anyone who could both demonstrate its use and also show you how to cultivate its acquisition in your practice. Master Wang could do that and insisted that you could do that too.

As is often written in books about tai chi, one of the outward illustrations of good chi development and chi circulation is a feeling of warmth and perhaps some "expansion" or "swelling" of the hands and fingertips. If such sensations result from your form practice, this is considered to be a good sign that you are on the right track.

In my form practice, it was probably longer than I care to admit before such sensations began to even sporadically occur. The odd thing about such episodes is that you can't seem to predict just when they will crop up. One day you will find your hands being warm and full and other days they will be cold, cold, cold. Sometimes during a single round of form, they will go from one extreme to another. On yet another day, the cycles might not swing so wildly. Some days there is no discernible difference whatsoever from start to finish.

What is a student/practitioner to make of all this? Nothing at all. That seems to be the best advice. The student should not be overly concerned one way or the other. Just continue practicing is what I've been told by more than one teacher whose opinion I respect and value. In due time, consistent daily practice will take you where you need to go.

Back to the story. During practice, Master Wang does not let his students don gloves at any time of the year. Coat, hat, scarf, yes; but, no gloves. On this particular Saturday morning, after we finished the second round of form, he called me over and asked me if my hands were warm. He *would frequently grab them to assess their temperature. This morning they were not warm. Had you been there, a nice, insulated, pair of gloves or simply putting your hands into your jacket pocket would've been your fondest wish. Although the wind was still, it was cold.*

"Watch", he said.

Master Wang then extended his arms slightly forward and closed both of his hands into the shape of a fist, palms up. Not a tightly clenched fist. Just the relaxed fist shape as you would make in the form. The tips of his finger pads were lightly touching the palm and the thumb placed nearby. After a few seconds, he slowly opened both hands. As he did so, steam-like vapors trailed lightly upward from the heart of his palms at the Lao Gong acupuncture point. It reminded me of tendrils arising from a warm cup of tea.

"Internal chi energy", he said and laughed. I just shook my head in acknowledgment.

We eventually went inside to our morning tea where I warmed my hands around the delicate cup and wondered about these things.

The next morning dawned equally cold. After our practice, he again demonstrated this remarkable phenomenon. My own hands did not follow his example that morning either.

Over the years I've seen him do this demonstration on several other occasions but that first time will always stick in my mind as a reminder of what is possible in this art.

More practice.

Ted

At the Antique Store
(Chapter 9: The Seven Principles of Tai Chi)

One Saturday, when I was invited up to Vancouver for a weekend visit with Master Wang, I drove us to an antique store that he wanted to visit. Truth be told, it wasn't so much an antique store as it was a second-hand furniture and bric-a-brac store. Upon entering, Master Wang and I greeted the Chinese owner and then he and I split up and began exploring. I'd been in many such stores with him and it quickly became apparent that this one contained one of the more unusual, incongruous, and eclectic collections we had come across. The inventory was a trifle eccentric.

Master Wang would sometimes spend more time examining things as he first came across them than I would. My general plan of attack was to survey an entire place and then take a second run at sections that I found interesting. On this day, I quickly worked my way through the merchandise and headed to the rear, right-hand section of the store while Master Wang was still up at the front.

As we'd entered, I noticed that this back corner was completely different from every other part of the store. A large area had been sort of fenced off with what I recall were low-standing bookcases. Inside the makeshift enclosure, a considerable number of wooden African sculptures had been amassed. Many of them were recognizable animal forms but some of them were human or quasi-human shapes. Some of the human sculptures were nearly life-size but most of the standing ones were probably only four or five feet tall, or perhaps even less. For the most part, they were crudely carved and certainly not well finished. Those that were not made of actual dark wood had been discolored with dye or perhaps burned with a blowtorch so that they had a scorched appearance. Some looked quite menacing while others were only slightly less so.

Apart from the images themselves and the considerable number amassed in such a small space, what was most striking about the whole collection was the faintly ominous atmosphere surrounding the assemblage. Although I consider myself a pretty rational person, I had the *thought and a gut feeling that this area was slightly threatening and "creepy", for lack of a better word. Having satisfied my initial curiosity, I found myself not wanting to linger there very long. So, I purposefully moved on and continued my exploration of what was turning out to be a rather large store.*

About twenty or thirty minutes later, I met up again with Master Wang at the front of the store. In a diagonal direction, we were about as far away from those African statues as you could be and still be in the building. As I recall, there were no other customers in the store just then nor had there been since we arrived. Although the owner greeted us when we entered, he then left us alone and went to attend to other business.

Master Wang motioned me closer and asked me to look at his hands. I didn't know what I was supposed to be looking for. Had he cut himself? Had he had an allergic reaction to something we'd eaten a little while before?

"Look at my fingertips.", he said.

Much to my surprise, his fingertips each had a large water blister on them. On both hands, the entire pad on the end of each finger was completely puffed up and filled with liquid, just like you might see after a bad burn or scalding. Perhaps the thumbs did too, although I can't accurately recall.

"What happened?", I asked.

"It's chi. I was looking around back in that corner where all those statues are stored together. My body had a spontaneous reaction to the severe imbalance and negative energy present there and my hands began to swell up like this. The energy there is all wrong.", he said.

Together, we again walked back to the rear corner of the store. Master Wang again remarked about the negative energy surrounding the vicinity. I told him I had had a similar feeling of the area being menacing and "creepy" but of course, I didn't have a physical reaction anything like his. We were only back in that corner briefly before he headed us elsewhere.

We continued to idle our way through the rest of the store until Master Wang decided he'd seen enough and then we left. As we were walking down the block to my car, he showed me his hands again. The swelling and blisters were all gone. You'd never have known they were there.

As we drove away, Master Wang explained that as a result of his tai chi practice, he had developed an increased level of sensitivity to the environment, to people, to works of art, and to feng shui in general. This sensitivity was heightened by his cultivation of chi and a type of sixth sense which allows him to immediately recognize and respond to energetic imbalance or unease.

Although now I am more familiar with the preventive and health-promoting benefits of having strong chi, to this day I don't fully understand what that episode with Master Wang's hands was all about.

Ted

Stand Up, Sit Down
(Chapter 13: "Search Center")

Master Wang is a Push Hands (tui shou) champion who does not teach Push Hands. He would prefer that his students not participate in any Push Hands practice. And, if they do participate in it, he would prefer that they confine themselves to "neutralizing" the attacks of others rather than trying to throw the opponent out. He is similarly opposed to student participation in Push Hands tournaments, at least those conducted under the current format and rules.

Instead of Push Hands, Master Wang teaches a method of partner-practice interaction he calls "Search Center". A student's introduction to "Search Center" work may often begin with some "couch time" with Master Wang while he "searches your center".

To begin, you face forward with your back to a couch if one is available, or to a chair or bench if there is no couch. You stand in the "bow stance/archer's stance", which is a common stance in tai chi and other martial arts as well. All your weight rests on just the back leg and foot (100/0). The front leg is "empty". Although the front foot is flat on the ground, it contains and supports no weight. You are "100% rooted" in your back leg and your task is to maintain your "root" and stay standing. Your hands are held outward, perhaps in a variation of the "Push" or "Lift Hands" posture.

Master Wang stands directly in front of you in a similar stance. His front foot and your front foot are on either side of an imaginary line. He puts his hands or a "ward off" arm out so that you can touch him. When you've made your initial contact with him, he will then make a slight movement and you will find yourself seated on the couch. You were not aware that any physical force was used to put you there. How did that happen?

You stand up and the cycle begins again. You resume your securely "rooted" posture on the back leg. You extend your hands toward Master Wang. You sit down on the couch.

You stand up again. This time you are determined that you will stand there longer. You make yourself stiffer or stronger to be better able to resist his gentle action. You try harder. As a result, you find yourself sitting down even quicker than before and with even more momentum. You are glad the couch is there to break your fall.

You pop up again for another go. This interaction gets repeated perhaps 10 or 12 times in a row. Always on the same "rooted" leg. The outcome is always the same. You are always getting up.

You now are instructed to "switch legs". The lead leg becomes the rear leg and the exercise continues anew. You stand there in your "root" with your weight entirely on the fresh, back leg. If you hadn't already been doing so, you begin to anticipate the line of his "attack" and try to wiggle one way or another to deflect or defeat it. You began your gyrations even as contact is made. You sit down.

You vary your tactics. This time you go "all jelly body", twisting this way and that to "yield and neutralize" the incoming energy. You find yourself seated again. Your evasion was ineffective.

Your legs are now burning from all the weight-bearing work and the constant getting up and down. You wish that the couch wasn't such a low one. On some occasions, you might be lucky enough to have someone take pity and stack a second cushion on top of the first. That way you don't have so far to travel on the increasingly exhausting rebound.

You are getting up a little more slowly each time. Your breathing has become a little labored. Your body is weary. Your enthusiasm for more one-on-one time with your sifu is dwindling. You begin to wish that it was the next person's turn so that you could take a little rest. You are tired of the fight and a little dispirited by the futility of your efforts to elude Master Wang's gentle invitation to "be seated".

Unaccountably, an old high school cheer runs through your head as you slowly get back up yet again:

"Swing to the left,
Swing to the right,
Stand up. Sit down.
Fight! Fight! Fight!"
You find yourself wondering if it is time for tea yet.

Ted

The Flannel Shirt Incident
(Chapter 14: "No Touch" Work)

One late fall weekend, my friend Neal and I were invited to visit Master Wang in Vancouver. Neal is a professional chef whom I'd met through Saul Krotki's tai chi class in Seattle. He had studied culinary arts in Paris and had worked in high-end kitchens around the world and throughout the United States. At that time, Neal was working as a sous chef in one of the fine-dining restaurants in Seattle. Eventually, he married and left to take a position with the Ritz Carlton hotels and resorts group.

Master Wang has always insisted that the soft way and the use of internal chi power was the hallmark of tai chi and what distinguished it from the hardstyle martial arts. Part and parcel of correct practice was the unification of the mind and body in the gathering and direction of this chi power. In his judgment, what was often overlooked in tai chi training was the active role of the mind.

He emphasized that soft power is best generated by combining one's focused attention with suitable intention. Like focusing the beam of a magnifying glass to start a fire, a concentrated mind is also essential to achieving a proper outward expression of the energy inherent in this internal martial art. He insisted that anyone could manifest this effect once they had developed the correct understanding.

On this occasion, eager to demonstrate his point, Master Wang had Neal and I line up facing each other. As Neal was the "junior" student at the moment, he positioned Neal in the tai chi stance with his back toward the couch (i.e., the "Archer's Stance" with feet shoulder-width apart, front foot pointed straight ahead, the rear foot turned outward at a forty-five-degree angle). Neal's task was to put 100% of his weight on his rear leg and keep the front leg touching the floor but without any weight on it. I stood opposite him, face to face, in the same basic stance with our front toes not crossing over an imaginary line on the floor.

That day I'd worn a flannel shirt over a polo shirt but had taken off the flannel because our earlier practice had warmed things up. Master Wang had me get the discarded, flannel shirt and instructed me to wind it up in a manner like you would use to wring out a wet towel. He then told me to hand one end of this twisted shirt to Neal while I held the other. So now, in effect, Neal and I had a makeshift flannel rope lightly stretched between us.

Next, Master Wang said to me, "Use your mind and extend your chi to make Neal sit down on the couch".

I thought he was either kidding or crazy. This made absolutely no sense. How was I going to use a twisted piece of cloth to force Neal to sit down? If I pushed on our improvised "rope" it would simply sag and collapse between us. If we'd been holding a broom handle or stick, I might have a chance (using physical force but "minimally" of course) but using a limp shirt was out of the question.

Master Wang saw my skeptical and puzzled expression.

"Just try", he said.

Neal was willing, so I tried. To this day, I am grateful that there was no camera. I'm sure my face was comically contorted as I strained to put as much concentration as I could bring to bear on this task. A task I'd already convinced myself was ridiculous and beyond doing. Not surprisingly, nothing happened on the first attempt.

"Try again.", sifu said.

And again. And again. And again, etc., etc. Try as I might, nothing happened. After each failed effort, I was getting progressively more annoyed. Annoyed at my ineptitude and even more annoyed at sifu's insistence that I keep repeating this laughable mission.

As my fruitless efforts continued, Master Wang would make a suggestion or offer a comment from time to time. The core instructions were for me to "relax" and "connect" to Neal and then "expand" the energy. What the hell was he talking about! My exasperation was growing, albeit silently, but certainly not unnoticed by sifu.

Then, all of a sudden, Neal bent at the waist as if in reaction to receiving a punch in the stomach and he sat right down on the couch. Both of us were stunned. Master Wang didn't seem at all surprised.

To this day, I'm not entirely convinced that Neal hadn't simply sat down because I'd burned out his rear leg and "root". After all, I'd kept him standing there in that one-legged posture, holding all his weight on just one foot, for several minutes as I struggled with the exercise.

Neal assured me several times that sitting down voluntarily was not what he'd done. He said that one minute he was just standing there and the next thing he knew he found himself on his way to sitting down. He maintained that it was the chi that moved him, which had been an entirely new sensation for him. If so, I had no real understanding of what I'd done or, more to the point, just how I'd managed to do it.

When Neal and I later tried to recreate the scenario during our practice sessions in Seattle, we weren't successful. Whether using a towel, sweatshirt, jacket, or some other item of apparel, neither one of us could do it to the other.

Perhaps I never should have washed that magic flannel shirt.

Ted

Use the Mind, Not Force
(Chapter 12: Transitions & The Chi Trail)

One of the training exercises that Master Wang has his students perform is "The Seated Pull". It involves sitting on a chair or bench and seeing if your partner can disturb your seated position by pulling steadily on your outstretched arm. The sitter positions his or her body on the front edge of the chair or bench with the sit bones near the edge. The back is vertical and the feet are flat on the ground about shoulder-width apart. The sitter extends an arm and the puller grasps the outstretched palm like executing a handshake. Sometimes the puller will use two hands, one in the handshake grip and the other grasping the sitter's wrist. Once the two people are attached in this manner, the puller begins to apply a slow but steadily increasing amount of pull on the sitter's arm in an effort to disturb the sitter's posture and perhaps even pull him or her up and out of the seated position. (See Appendix C for a more detailed explanation of "The Seated Pull" exercise.)

So that is how the basic "The Seated Pull" exercise is performed. But what I wanted to talk about here is the next level of practice. Or, what occurred on this one particular evening.

As I remember it, Master Wang's house in Vancouver had an "open" floor plan in the area between the family room and the kitchen. There was no wall separating the two spaces. Although it contained a couple of comfortable leather couches and an end table, this area was intentionally left free of more furniture so that tai chi practice could be conducted indoors if needed.

One weekend, I arrived to find that he had installed a beautiful hardwood floor in the family room. To protect the new floor from scratches, the bottom of each leg of the dining table and chairs had been fitted with little, stick-on, felt pads. When the chairs were pulled away from the table, the pads allowed them to slide smoothly across the floor.

A couple of other students and I were there but memory escapes me as to those in attendance. We were discussing the importance of mental focus and the use of the mind (Yi) in tai chi practice. One of Master Wang's Seven Principles is "Concentration". Oversimplified, the rule requires that while engaging in tai chi practice the mind must remain "focused" on the task at hand and cannot be allowed to drift away or become inattentive, even for an instant.

Master Wang said that in practicing the tai chi form in this manner you would experience the power of thought and its effects on the body's response to its environment. The mind/body connection is something of considerable interest these days in the sciences. Even in the popular press, there are more and more references to new findings concerning this dynamic interplay.

So, as part of this evening's discussion, I find myself in the role of the sitter in "The Seated Pull" exercise. I'm poised on the edge of the dining room chair with my stockinged feet planted on the slippery floor. Despite the felt pads on the chair legs, I'd been able so far to withstand the persistence of the puller during a few attempts. Then the rules of the game were changed.

Master Wang directed me to pick my feet up off the ground and hook them around the chair legs so they wouldn't be touching the floor. Which I do. Then he has the puller grab my extended arm just as before and pull. (Was it my chef friend Neal? I don't remember.) After some initial inertia, the chair and I glide smoothly in the direction of the pull. Of course. Just what you'd expect.

Then Master Wang said that I should now ignore the pull on my arm and instead concentrate my mind exclusively on the idea of "down" or "sinking my Center (lower dan tien) into the floor and ground". I think to myself that this instruction is ridiculous and will be completely ineffectual, not to mention potentially embarrassing to me but entertaining to the audience on hand. So, as I wonder how I'm supposed to ignore a pull that I certainly feel and whose effects I've already experienced, I try to focus my mind as he'd instructed.

I focus, the puller pulls and the chair and I glide smoothly forward.

"Do it again and focus this time", Master Wang says.

Once more and the chair still slides but it takes a little while longer. Hmm?

"Again", sifu directs.

At this point, I'm nearly breaking a sweat as I'm trying to concentrate as hard as I can. I'm sure my brow is furrowed and that my body has tensed up too. We've all seen little kids grip their pencils tighter when trying to print their names. Sometimes they even extend their tongues in some tortured shape to aid the tip of the pencil along its path. As if tensing the body would help the mind's powers to focus. Oh well. I resolved to do the opposite. Relax and focus.

This time the chair does not move. The puller is fully engaged but the chair and I remain stationary. Suddenly aware of its immobility, I break concentration to marvel at that fact, and the chair and I immediately begin to slide.

"Do it again". This time it is me, not Master Wang, requesting the puller to grab my arm. He does. I focus. I don't look at him. I don't look at anyone in the room. I am aware of the pulling sensation on my arm but I focus only on the idea of "down". The puller relaxes and I realize that I remain where we started. The chair has not moved.

Beginner's luck?

Ted

"Yong Yi, Bu Yong Li"

◆ ◆ ◆

Resources

Master Henry Wang's Website:
www.searchcentertaichi.com

Master Henry Wang's Facebook Page:
https://www.facebook.com/MasterHenryWang/

YouTube Videos. Enter search terms:
"Master Henry Wang" or "Master Henry Wang Tai Chi"

Contact Information:
Master Henry Wang
2133 Downey Ave.
Comox, B.C., V9M 1W7
Canada

Email: hiwangtaichi@telus.net

◆ ◆ ◆

About the Author

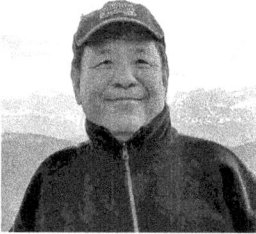

Master Henry Wang (Wang, Hui-Juin) was born in Taiwan. He lived there until 1987 when he and his family immigrated to British Columbia, Canada. He is married to Ivy. They have two adult children and three grandchildren. Master Wang and Ivy live on Vancouver Island, in the town of Comox, British Columbia. Master Wang has devoted over forty-five years to the study, practice, and teaching of Tai Chi Chuan.

About the Co-Author

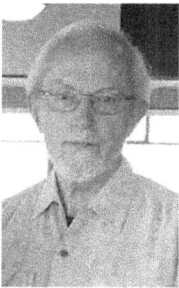

Ted Libby is originally from Detroit, Michigan. He moved to Seattle in 1992 and started taking tai chi classes there in 1993. Ted has studied with Master Wang since 1997 and began teaching tai chi classes in 2008. He teaches in Issaquah, Washington, a suburb located east of Seattle in the foothills of the Cascade Range. His practice group is named after Tiger Mountain, one of the five "Issaquah Alps".

https://tigermountaintaichi.com

♦ ♦ ♦

Postscript re Collaboration

Writing this book has been a truly collaborative enterprise undertaken by a tai chi master and one of his many students.

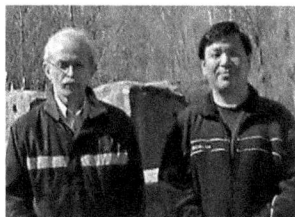

At Master Wang's suggestion and with his encouragement, it began with a series of in-person, free-ranging, audiotape conversations between Master Wang and myself during my irregular visits to Vancouver, B.C.

Between visits, I transcribed and organized each session under various topics. After that, I would call Master Wang to discuss the latest transcript and would offer my suggestions and comments from a student's perspective. Where appropriate, he would then provide more detailed explanations and clarifications. Often, he would add new topics and other subject matter as well.

This review process resulted in my taking further notes during our intermittent, extended telephone conversations. Those notes, on both the old and new material, were then added to the relevant topics. As the project continued to grow, a series of draft manuscripts were prepared, revised, and reorganized as a consequence of our additional ongoing conversations. Meetings followed with Master Wang in Vancouver and Comox, British Columbia to review and discuss particular drafts. Ultimately, the project was completed.

Based on over forty-five years of devoted study and practice, this final version is a chronicle of Master Wang's experiences, insights, and teachings. To the extent that there are factual errors or other misstatements, the mistakes are surely mine.

For a variety of reasons related to my schedule and the process involved, the project took longer to complete than either of us expected. Nevertheless, as Master Wang has pointed out to me, "The turtle wins the race."

Ted

Co-Author's Acknowledgments

I would like to thank Master Wang and the many other people who have supported this undertaking.

Several friends read through successive drafts of various chapters and to them I am particularly grateful. Special thanks and appreciation to Joe Zanbilowicz for reviewing the final manuscript with Master Wang and for his patient examination and thoughtful suggestions regarding final edits. Similar recognition should also be extended to Peter Uhlmann, Mo MacKendrick, and Greg Harley who provided helpful comments on earlier drafts.

Thanks also to the following senior students for their contributions concerning their experiences with Master Wang, namely: Chris Bryhan, Greg Harley, Tak J. Kong, Summer McGee, James Milne, Lawrie Milne (no relation), Dennis Peska, Paul Seronko, Peter Uhlmann, Ann Zanbilowicz, and Joe Zanbilowicz.

I likewise want to express my appreciation to Master Wang's Canadian students for their warm welcome, fellowship, and gracious hospitality over the years at Master Wang's annual summer camps, workshops, and other get-togethers.

In addition to my studies with Master Wang and his wife, Ivy, who is an accomplished watercolor artist and a much-appreciated tai chi teacher in her own right, I have had the great good fortune in my tai chi life to have studied with other highly accomplished and dedicated teachers from the Cheng Man-ch'ing lineage. In particular, I want to express my appreciation and gratitude to Saul Krotki and my classmates in his Bear Palm Tai Chi Association, Seattle, Washington. For the past twenty-five years, Saul has led us in the faithful and spirited practice of the Professor's tai chi form, sword form, and Push Hands.

Similar thanks to Carol Yamasaki (1944-2021), Bret Hall, and Carol's other students who also carefully preserve and study the Professor's lessons in Birmingham, Michigan. For many years, Carol, my friend and teacher, and her entire group have cordially welcomed me to their practices during my annual winter holiday visits with my sisters in Michigan. Sadly, the lineage has now lost another respected teacher; Carol died peacefully at home on April 7, 2021.

A debt of gratitude is also owed to the late David C. Chen (1955-2005), and his widow, Joanne C. Chang, for their many kindnesses and gracious hospitality while I attended classes at their Wu Wei Tai Chi Club, Rockville, Maryland. Thanks also to the late Dr. Tao, Ping Siang (1919-2006), and the Five Willow Tai Chi Association, Seattle, Washington where I first learned the Cheng, Man-ch'ing tai chi form.

Thanks too for all I have learned from the students, past and present, in my classes at Tiger Mountain Tai Chi Chuan, Issaquah, Washington during the past twelve years.

Special thanks to Chris Bryhan and Simon Leon, fellow teachers and colleagues, for their dedication to "Search Center" practice and to Bryan Ellis for his friendship and encouragement throughout.

Finally, I also want to thank the Temple Ratz, a truly undisciplined, Monday night practice group, for their friendship and many a noteworthy, post-practice dinner outing to the remarkable Chinese restaurants in Seattle's International District.

Master Wang would say it is karma.

Ted Libby

♦ ♦ ♦

www.ingramcontent.com/pod-product-compliance
Lightning Source LLC
Chambersburg PA
CBHW071644310326
41914CB00128B/2058/J